PRAIS
FROM FA7

"WOW! The book made me feel like I could be successful at not only weight loss but also at loving myself. I will absolutely recommend this book to others. I just must know—did you like the hard-boiled egg? I also like the "Then what?" question game. You, my dear, will change lives because of your book. Thank you for giving me the opportunity to read it."

— Ronda DeLaughter

"Thank you for all you are doing to help people get healthy and take back their lives!"

— Carrie Boeser

"I will be forever grateful to you for all of your transparency, sharing your pain, and how you deal with normal life. I feel like I've been thrown a lifeline."

— Gina Hall

"I just wanted to say thank you! Some of my favorite [parts] are What If? and Fear Is A Liar. You are smart, funny, relatable, and humble/down to earth! Thank you for being you and speaking straight from the heart! You are a blessing to many in this journey/lifestyle!"

— Christina Leilua

"Gosh, I relate to this so much...like so, so much. I have never heard anyone like me. I am the biggest emotional eater. I hate it and beat myself up every day. Thank you."

— Dezaray VanTrup

"Thank you for sharing with all of us! This is so spot-on for me, with my life right now. Facing a possible career change, my current company asking me, 'What do we have to do to keep you?' Fear!! You have given me a part of the confidence that is missing in my life. Thank you, thank you for all the positive, amazing advice!"

— Aubrey Heinzelman

"Elizabeth's teachings on overcoming emotional eating have been such a blessing to me. She is so transparent with her own struggles with emotional eating that it makes her message even more relatable and impactful! Her encouragement has led me to dig deep and tackle many of these issues that I have struggled with for decades."

— Sarah Cunningham

A GIFT FOR YOU:
FROM FAT TO FREE
ACTION PLAN JOURNAL

Get the PDF version of the action plan companion journal to *From Fat To Free* for free.

Are you ready to end your toxic relationship with food?

To access your gift...

1. Visit https://www.FromFattoFree.com/freegift.

2. Tell us where to email your access link.

3. Check your email to download your journal.

4. As you read this book, follow along using the journal to complete activities and make notes.

from fat to free

How to End Your Toxic Relationship with Food

ELIZABETH LIZBERG

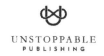

UNSTOPPABLE
PUBLISHING

Library of Congress Control Number: 2020920656

Print ISBN: 978-1-7358589-0-6

E-book ISBN: 978-1-7358589-1-3

Unstoppable Publishing
231 Public Square, Suite 300
Franklin, Tennessee 37064

Editing by Julie Willson

Cover Design by Sophia Lizberg and Carew Co.

Interior Layout by Janell E. Robisch, Speculations Editing

Photography by Erin Blackwell Studios

DISCLAIMER

The content provided in this book is designed to supply helpful information on the subjects discussed. This book is not meant to be used, nor should it be used, to diagnose or treat any medical condition. For diagnosis or treatment of any medical problem, consult your own physician. The publisher and the author are not responsible for any specific health or allergy needs that may require medical supervision, and are not liable for any damages or negative consequences for any treatment, action, application, or preparation to any person reading or following the information in this book. References are provided for informational purposes only and don't constitute endorsement of any websites or other sources. Readers should also be aware that the websites listed in this book may change or become obsolete.

This book is dedicated to those who came, saw, and stayed.

Unconditional love forever to

Mom, Dad, John, Ted

Kim and my sweet nieces, Bella and Aubrey

Bonus children Kenny and Katie

Sophie—my love, my life

CONTENTS

INTRODUCTION

Are you screaming from the inside? Do you know that you're living a life that's not what you actually want? You know that something is supposed to be different, but you just keep finding yourself back at square one. It's not from lack of desire and certainly not from a lack of effort. You make changes with great intentions, but never get the results you're looking for. Why?

As I sit and write this to you, I am experiencing a new and different life every day. All of it reflects where I wanted to be when I was screaming from the inside, like you may be. Where did I want to be? What was I screaming for? My life is fulfilling and full of love. I enjoy waking up each day to see what is going to happen.

Did losing weight change all of this? No—I did! Forget being humble, it's the truth. Going from fat to free requires more than just learning how to use food to fuel your body. You've got to end the toxic relationship you have with food first. No person, no diet, and no industry can do that for you. You have to do the work.

If you're anything like I was, you probably don't believe it's possible. But I'm here to tell you that it is. You can lose the weight and keep it off.

After 35 years of battling being fat and trying nearly everything, I realized there was a key piece missing in all my efforts. I chose the Code Red Lifestyle (www.CodeRedLifestyle.com) to learn how to fuel my body appropriately. For the first time, I found a community of support and a formula that worked. But I also realized my relationship with food was far beyond fueling my body properly. My journey to climb this weight-loss mountain for the last time required me to address my toxic relationship with food.

Ending that relationship is what led me here, sharing my journey with you. I quickly discovered that there was no single resource available to sum up everything I needed to learn and address. There are many organizations that understand addiction. There are oodles of resources about changing habits, facing fears, adjusting your mindset, and learning how to love yourself. But none of them were assembled and outlined in a resource to guide or support me through it.

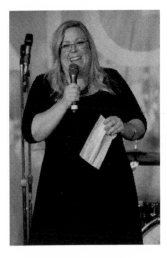 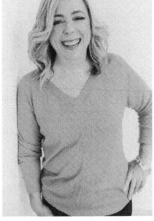

Me 2016   *Me 2020*

If you haven't determined how you'll learn to fuel your body, you need to. You must learn how to eat in a manner that doesn't leave you feeling hungry. And it needs to be sustainable. Code Red is what worked for me. There I found a level of support and education unlike any of the many diet plans I had tried. One of the major differences between this and other options is that you are taught to change your lifestyle and not just temporarily eat differently.

There are endless options out there for you. Be mindful about gimmicks and suggestions that don't include eating real food and reducing your sugar intake, or programs that insist you must buy their products in order to fuel your body.

Ultimately, my success came from both learning how to eat better and finding tools to end my toxic relationship with food. I recommend doing both at the same time. The inspiration derived from a dropping number on the scale is helpful when you're vulnerable and learning how to navigate emotions you stuffed away a long time ago. The joy you experience when you have control over food—rather than it controlling you—will keep you strong when your body is not losing weight the way you want.

Most people don't want to talk about fat. There is so much shame and guilt around living life overweight. The word *fat* itself is offensive to many. The reality is, if we could deal with feelings and emotions in a more direct manner, we would have fewer people using food to fill their emotional needs rather than to simply fuel their bodies. If there was less personal shame and guilt and more education and resources, many of us would have a different relationship with food.

The food and health industries have more responsibility in this epidemic than anyone will acknowledge because of the power of money. But until the day comes when we can change the industry, we will all have to start with the one item we can control—ourselves.

This book was developed from journals I kept through many years of pain and struggles. It chronicles my experience taking off my fat armor and ending my toxic relationship with food. I fumbled through to find the resources I needed in order to take difficult steps. Fixing my outside didn't fix my insides. I believed for a long time that my fat was protecting me. But I found a way to let go. I can now protect myself when I need to, and I can also live free.

This book is filled with advice from my own experience. In my journey, I struggled to find others who understood my struggles and my desire to change until I started talking about it. Then I realized that thousands of others felt the same way I did.

> *Join my Facebook page (<u>From Fat To Free</u>) and you'll be surrounded by people who understand.*

The challenge and success of my journey has inspired me to tell my story in the hope that it will provide enlightenment, inspire action, and lead you to experience the joy of going from fat to free.

Your resources to get you started are in this book. The tools I developed (and still use today) are all provided. But there is work to be done, and you must be willing to do it. I've included several take action activities throughout this book. Use the companion *From Fat To Free Action Plan Journal* to follow along with the chapters, complete additional exercises, and find inspiration. If you don't have this resource, get yourself a nice journal and pen and keep them with this book.

This will be hard, but I promise you it will be worth it. Life doesn't get easier; you get stronger.

It's time to live the life you've imagined. Are you ready? I know the answer. The real question is...

Are you willing?

SETTING THE STAGE

FAT: JANUARY 16, 2006

I will be 36 this year, and I still hide behind my fat. I have yet to have a real connection with anyone. I am tired of being lonely, but I continue to make choices that help me avoid living. I have a great life with [my daughter] Sophie, but cringe at the thought of what I am teaching her. I see her learning how to hide and to be scared of what the world offers. Rather than truly feeling all of this, I eat.

A SOUTHERN PEACH

I loved my home in Atlanta, Georgia. Brooklawn Road. We had THE BEST backyard. It was full of tall trees, with an amazing treehouse my dad built. Behind our house was a creek where we would spend hours each day looking for tadpoles or dangling over the water on our tire swing. Our neighborhood group of kids played through elementary years and started teen years together. My earliest memories are slip-and-slides on the front lawn, climbing trees, swimming, and bike riding until the streetlights would come on and tell us it was time to head home. That house witnessed so many of my firsts—my first dog, my first bike, my first kiss.

Growing up in Georgia, I was a southern peach. I knew how to properly entertain, write thank-you notes, and even how to iron bedsheets. My dad worked and my mom was home with us. My two brothers, John and Ted, kept their brotherly harassment to a minimum and always made it known that they had my back. My family (by blood or by choice) has always been a priority and a constant in my life, and I credit them for many of my blessings today.

Despite growing up in this idyllic setting, I started to view my body in a negative light. When I was younger, I never paid attention because I was comfortable. I was active. I played soccer and ran track and cross country. We rode our bikes every day. I felt good. I remember being happy.

When I was in eighth grade, my parents transferred me to a different school. I wasn't pleased about leaving my friends and starting something new. From an early age, I always reacted to change with a high level of dramatics. My brother Ted had already been at the new school for a year, so I found comfort in his experience and willingness to introduce me to new friends, and I started to settle in.

One day while walking down the hall, I overheard a boy (you know the one—the popular one) say to my newest friend, "I don't want her to come to my party. She's a beached whale." OUCH!

And so the seed was planted. My negative self-image started spiraling. How could I be comfortable knowing that's what people thought of me? My middle school years continued with more of the same awkward and hurtful situations. I truly felt alone. As children, we are not able to see when others feel awkward. We're all just trying to figure out how to feel accepted and loved ourselves.

A BIG CHANGE

Our house at Brooklawn Road was my home until the day my parents announced we were moving to Boise, Idaho. I was shocked and devastated. (Remember, change for me equals drama.) How could Idaho ever compare to everything I knew in Georgia? We were moving from the city to the country, from shopping malls and hair salons to cowboy boots and rodeos. All I knew about Idaho was potatoes. My mind began drafting an emotional, sensational story of what was to come. (What teen wouldn't be concerned when her shopping habit was going from a four-story mall to no mall at all!)

My parents said it would be an adventure filled with new opportunities. They promised blue skies and mountains unlike anything I had ever seen. I could start driving at the age of 14, plus there would be no traffic or long commutes to school. They said it was an opportunity for a better life, but I didn't understand at the time. A big change was happening, whether I liked it or not.

We had going-away parties and laughed at gifts of cowboy boots, candy bars shaped like potatoes, and jokes about wearing Levi's 501 jeans (which in Atlanta were only mentioned in farming commercials). My mom worked hard to celebrate a new home, new friends, and a new school. At times, she inspired excitement, intrigue, and curiosity in me. But nothing calmed the anger I felt over my lack of control. I was terrified of change.

But eventually the moving trucks came and packed up my last 13 years. The house was empty, but my heart was full of memories I'd hold on to forever.

When our plane took off, my mom started sobbing. She was worried they had made the wrong decision. I didn't realize it at the time, but she had been the strong one through the announcement and all the planning surrounding the move. She had been hiding her emotions and fears about the impact of this decision on us kids and our family. She could no longer hold it in.

I don't remember the details of *why* my mom had to end up using a bra as a tissue to wipe her face, but I do remember that the absurdity of the moment moved us all from tears to laughter. At that moment, we turned a corner and started to look toward the future.

FITTING IN

Idaho was definitely an adjustment. It took years to understand why my parents had made such a drastic move, but I grew to love this state. (And Boise later got a mall, so that helped.) But at 13, I felt like I was starting all over again. Everything felt awkward. I spoke funny. I now had to drink "pop" instead of "Coke" (the universal name for all sodas in Georgia). Levi's were more than just commercials and "y'all" was quickly correcting to "you guys." I was observing and adjusting. I was abandoning preferences I had known all my life so I could try to fit in.

But changing the way I spoke wasn't enough to disappear into the crowd. By high school, I felt an intense pressure to be skinnier. I wasn't medically overweight, but I was certainly bigger than my friends. I referred to myself as "mushy." An early example of how I protected myself through humor. If I made jokes about myself so others laughed, maybe they would look past my insecurities and the fact that my body was different than theirs.

I had a loving mother who often cooked for us—good southern cooking that was always plentiful. One of her greatest pleasures was to spend the day creating snacks for us to eat after school. The foods I now refer to as "junk" were always accessible.

She also helped us cope with difficult times by feeding us. One time she told me that the best part of her day was preparing all sorts of snacks for us to choose from when we got home from school. I remember walking in the house to a fridge and freezer full of treats.

She always cooked though. Never bought the boxed or processed foods, as they were not good for us. It didn't matter what emotion was going on, there was always food...good food. I mean, we were from the South, the birthplace of "comfort food." Eating to comfort sadness, eating to celebrate success, or eating to calm our anger. It was commonplace, and when combined with the addictive nature of sugar, these were key ingredients in a recipe that made me fat for many years.

As peer pressure increased, I tried to find ways to lose the fat. At the time, "fat-free" was the recommendation for weight loss. I remember shopping with my mom and believing we could eat cookies and chips and drink pop because they didn't have fat. (It's shocking to me now how drastically we lost the simplest idea: eat real food.)

I believe these trendy messages played a significant role in my ride on the diet merry-go-round. Food industries continue to adapt to the latest fads and spend millions of dollars to market the latest craze to those of us desperate to get the weight off. My attempts to lose weight with these fads were the same as many—Weight Watchers, shakes, and pills. I even considered the drastic measure of gastric bypass surgery. But none of it addressed the real problem.

High school was four more years of trying to feel accepted and loved by other people. I often heard, "You need to love yourself first," but at the time I didn't understand what it meant or why it was essential. By college, I had created a life consumed with what others thought and felt about me. I thought the best way to gain acceptance and love was by doing whatever made other people happy. I was a pleaser.

This desire to please others carried on throughout my life, and with it, my body got bigger, my health got worse, and my self-worth sunk lower. (I have years of journals with the same underlying premise: my lack of self-worth, the struggles of being a victim, and my efforts to appease everyone but myself.)

I got married, had a child, got divorced, became a single parent, went back to college, and found a solid professional career—but the fundamental theme of my stories never changed. More and more, food became my comfort. Food was my friend and my support. It soothed me when times were hard. Like with any addiction, I needed it to feel protected.

BUILDING MY ARMOR

My memories of eating and hiding food go all the way back to Georgia. Food helped me feel in control. My days consisted of eating breakfast with my family and then stopping at a fast food restaurant or a gas station on the way to work. I'd buy several breakfast sandwiches, the largest pop they sold, and candy bars—all to consume before work. Before I could even finish all of that, I was thinking about where my next meal would come from, and this would continue throughout the day.

Dinner was almost always going to a restaurant or ordering takeout. When I was a single parent, any dinner at home was frequently served while watching television—in two separate rooms. Eating out was my preference because it always allowed for more food. Nobody questions you at a restaurant ordering drinks, appetizers, salads, a main course with two sides...and don't forget dessert!

I claimed that I didn't like fast food so we could go somewhere and sit down for a whole meal. When fast food was the only option, my preference was to go to the drive-thru and order as if I were feeding a large family. I'd say, "What does he want? I can't remember," and then proceed to order enough food for an entire family, which I ate in the parking lot. At other times, when shame and fear of judgment was more than I could overcome, I'd either go to several drive-thru windows or buy groceries in addition to fast food. If I was picking up dinner for the family, I'd order extra and eat it before getting home to sit at the dinner table and eat (again) with the family.

(I told you my identity was entirely rolled up in what other people thought of me. I have to roll my eyes now wondering what on earth made me think teenagers working at a fast-food joint cared even a little bit about what I ordered or who was eating it.)

Work wasn't any different for me, except my addiction was harder to hide. In stressful situations, I'd walk around the office scavenging. Many times, I'd declare, "I need..." then name my food of choice depending on the emotions I was experiencing. Usually it was chocolate, but the higher the stress level, the more substantial the choices—pizza, french fries, pasta.

During coworkers' birthdays, promotions, showers, or farewells, I'd enjoy treats with my office mates but miss the act of any camaraderie because I spent the whole time plotting how I'd be able to get more food without judgment. After the party had dispersed, I'd often return to the break room to indulge further.

This daily level of destruction, all in the name of protecting myself, led to many years of extreme loneliness. I developed a fear of real, true intimacy. While my journals will tell you I was desperate for a "real relationship," my fat was the ultimate shield. My shame and fear of rejection overpowered any attempt at a real connection. I couldn't develop true, honest relationships with friends or coworkers when I was trying so hard to hide so much of myself. I spent many years working to feel the love I so deeply desired, but also damaging my body so badly, leaving nothing but illness and despair.

ADD IN A VICTIM IDENTITY

My addiction continued to develop steadily over many years. I cultivated a fear of intimacy. I sank into a victim mindset. Nothing was my fault or within my control. Every challenge meant that life was unfair.

Life *was* unfair when my daughter was born weighing only 2.3 pounds. Nothing was normal about my pregnancy from the beginning. When I was in the middle of it, I chalked it up to another unfair situation and never connected it to my poor health.

We had been told that I would likely not get pregnant due to endometriosis and fibroid tumors. Well, what a blessing that they were wrong. One try and I was seeing double lines on the pregnancy stick.

My pregnancy was difficult medically, and around the same time, my marriage took a severe turn for the worse that resulted in a separation, so I was living with my parents.

My fibroid tumors landed me on bed rest, and at 29 weeks my blood pressure put me in the hospital. I was told it would be for one day to get my body under control, but it quickly became obvious that I would not be leaving anytime soon. My kidneys were damaged and would require additional surgery after my daughter was born.

I was determined to make it to term (which I now realize was a ridiculous notion). The doctors claimed I was "allergic" to pregnancy. I now believe that was their way to avoid saying that it was due to all the damage my obesity had done to my body over the years.

I was monitored closely with bloodwork and ultrasounds every day to check on our baby girl. I remember the day that my lifelong friend Jamie was with me at the ultrasound and the doctor declared, "It's time." I had no idea what he meant, but it didn't take long for the reality of the situation to set in. My placenta had broken down and was no longer providing her with what she needed in my womb. It was time for her to come out.

But it was too early. Babies need more than 30 weeks to develop. I had never felt her move or kick. I would not know the experience of childbirth. I had already failed as a mom and she wasn't even here yet. You can bet that led to some emotional eating.

Finally, Sophie arrived. She was a fighter from day one. She stayed in the hospital for 10 weeks of care and I was by her side every single day, all day. I was so scared.

You see, denial only goes so deep. I knew the truth. Denial and eating to numb the pain were so much easier than acknowledging my truth. (The good news is that she has grown up to be a beautiful, healthy, intelligent, sassy, fun, and loving young lady.)

Life was also unfair when I had to have a hysterectomy. Every failed relationship, night of loneliness, even mundane challenges like a flat tire meant my life was obviously so much harder than anyone else's.

I was killing myself emotionally and physically. My body was mere weeks away from requiring insulin. I was treating my Type 2 diabetes and high blood pressure with six different medications. My kidneys had suffered greatly during my pregnancy and continued to fail afterward. My doctor prepared me for the possibility of future dialysis. I broke bones in my feet due to the lack of feeling I had in them.

Diabetes is a slow progression of your body not functioning well. Neuropathy is one side effect, where you begin to lose feeling in your limbs. My hands were never impacted but my feet were, and at times my toes still tingle. My vision was steadily getting worse. I had no energy. My family noted how often I'd yawn. I was exhausted by midafternoon every day. I snored, and sleep was never restful.

Walking steps or hills was painful and embarrassing. I avoided small spaces and entered rooms wondering if I'd be the fattest one there. I dreaded shopping and feared anything new. I'd be surrounded by loved ones yet still feel empty and alone. I lived a life of lies and so desperately wanted something different. I hurt in every possible way. And watching my daughter follow in my footsteps was excruciating.

All this combined only fueled my choice to eat more, to try to mask the pain. The cycle was frustrating and discouraging. I was told to eat less and exercise. I heard endless advice without any substance. It was maddening and only served as evidence that others did not and could not understand what I was feeling.

I put on a brave face. I never asked for help or genuinely opened up to others. I could show no signs of weakness, and my only badge of success was that I tackled this life on my own.

BECOMING STRONG AND FREE

I was a strong woman. I did arduous things. I had many successes and moments of great joy. I have beautiful memories with family, friends, loved ones, and my daughter. I just did it all within an armor of fat. I had convinced myself that the fat was protecting me from pain and rejection. In reality, it was killing both my spirit and my body.

So I get every painful step you've taken.

I also get....

- ◇ Every cry in the shower, every hidden meal, every stuffing down of feelings.
- ◇ Walking into a room and wondering if you'll be the largest person there.
- ◇ Sitting in a chair and wondering whether it will break, not being able to squeeze into your car because the one next to you parked so close, avoiding mirrors because you can't stand to see what you think is a disgusting blob.
- ◇ Not being able to cross your legs or get to your seat in the middle of a theater row without asking everyone to stand up.
- ◇ Shopping and feeling like everything is a tent, sweating all the time, being out of breath and unable to participate in so much of life.
- ◇ Eating your food, your child's food, and any other food you can find (including old Halloween candy).

◇ Wondering whether this will be the meal that will cause your heart attack.

◇ Wondering whether you're going to feel alone forever.

◇ Every moment of regret as you watch life from a place of fear and loneliness with a brave face pasted on.

◇ Overcompensating in so many aspects of life, hoping you have some worth.

◇ Feeling worthless.

◇ What it feels like for the fat on your body to be so much heavier than just the pounds.

◇ What it's like to feel like your body is shutting down, and going to bed at the end of the day wondering whether you'll wake up the next morning.

I get what it feels like to be fat.

But now, I get what it's like to live FREE. And instead of being forced to deal with an imperfect and frustrating situation, I am now able to celebrate so many successes.

Here's what I get now...

◇ Having energy unlike anything I had before.

◇ Controlling how I fuel my body.

◇ Walking into a room with authentic confidence.

◇ Feeling emotions rather than stuffing them down with food.

◇ Moving without pain.

◇ What it's like to feel my feet again.

◇ Staring at my shadow in disbelief that it's so small, doing a double take in the mirror.

◇ No longer hiding from the camera.

◇ Tying my shoes without being out of breath.

◇ Shopping in any store without wondering whether they will carry my size.

◇ Being picky about dating, about what I want and not just what I have to settle for.

◇ Walking into work meetings and focusing on the topic at hand instead of whether they think I'm "less than" because I'm fat.

◇ Looking others in the eye and smiling without fear of the attention it may bring.

◇ Starting up conversations with strangers.

◇ Trying new skills—even scary activities like zip-lining and horseback riding. And fitting on all the rides at the fair.

◇ Only having to see doctors once a year.

◇ Spending hours doing activities that bring me joy. I don't have to feel selfish when I care for myself or make myself a priority.

◇ Looking in the mirror and saying, "I love you" without an ounce of doubt.

◇ Sharing my story and helping others on their journeys.

I get what it's like to live free.

FREE: JUNE 15, 2019

I keep secretly hoping that what I have learned will change. I want life challenges to go away. They won't. It's hard. Stay focused. Loving myself will by far be the greater gift than trying to make someone love me who doesn't. I am enough. I do hard things. I get to define my life and my worth.

FAT TO FREE ACTION PLAN

What is your story? Write the good, bad, sad, and most importantly the amazing!

You are going to be asked to dig deep in this process, and the next chapter will help you determine your inspiration when you are struggling.

CHAPTER ONE:
FINDING YOUR WHY

FAT: FEBRUARY 9, 2006

I don't like myself. I give up as soon as I get scared. What makes me even more unhappy is seeing myself in Sophie, then I get frustrated with her.

MY LIGHT BULB MOMENT

My "why" can be summed up in one word: Sophie. My daughter is my inspiration, my drive, my love, and my life. I had years of struggles, bad decisions, and life challenges. But I also found a lot of love, hope, and joy through her. My why is wanting even more of those great experiences with her.

I wrote the journal entry above when Sophie was six years old. It brings me back to a time when I was just going through the motions to get through each day. My joy in life was her, but at the same time, I was also heavy with regret, shame, and guilt from my choices and my parenting. I started to see Sophie develop some of the same traits I hated in myself. Fear was at the top of the list.

I remember many examples of my frustration being over the top because she would not try something new. One story that comes to mind was the hot summer day that I put a hose on her slide to help cool her off. I encouraged her to give it a try. She would not. As with most of my examples, my frustration was not warranted. It wasn't about her.

In reality, I was never mad at Sophie. The truth was that I saw the fear in her. I was frustrated that the only way she knew to face fear—the way I had taught her—was to back down and not try anything new, even something as simple as going down the slide.

We all have those moments we wish we could go back and change. For years, I had taught Sophie the exact behaviors I despised in myself. And I had no idea how to change. My reaction in that moment only added to her fear. My response was about me, but I took it all out on her because I was so afraid she would turn out to be just like me.

Sophie has always been my primary why, but many heart-aches contributed to the decision to finally change my life. My body was quitting on me. I had witnessed loved ones suffer during their own health challenges. I was in a relationship but still felt alone. I watched my daughter turn to food after struggling with some typical teenage-friendship issues.

Eventually, the light bulb came on. By that time, Sophie was going to leave for college soon, and I had only a brief time to teach her how to respond to life's challenges without involving food. I desperately wanted her to avoid living a fat life and experiencing all the disappointments that come with it. I was determined to send her off armed with the knowledge to make good choices. She was my driving force.

REALITY HITS

I finally started learning how to fuel my body, and my family became interested in getting healthy as well. Sophie started noticing when she dealt with challenges by turning to food and gradually learned to make better choices. It felt good to share my reality with others; it felt even better to see my daughter take interest in learning how to fuel her body properly. We were all working together and feeling more confident each day.

By this point, I had lost 70 pounds. However, I was naïve in thinking that weight loss would solve everything. Life happened, and I began to realize how much work was still ahead of me.

For a year, Sophie and I struggled with the emotions and challenges of her dad being extremely sick. Her dad, Tim, battled his own addictions with food and alcohol. We had many issues that led us down the path of divorce by the time our daughter was two. One of the most common fights was my concern for him being an alcoholic. He assured me, to the point of great anger, that I was wrong. We went our separate ways and I figured I had it all wrong.

I never spoke of it again until the final year of his life. We lived in different states, so I didn't know that he had been drinking every day since our divorce. That year, Sophie and I watched him struggle with the disease and our hearts hurt because we couldn't help him. We knew it was bad, but were in denial about how bad. Or maybe we just didn't want to feel that pain.

Eventually, the call came. Within two hours, my daughter and I were on a plane to say goodbye. It is hard to find the words to describe the pain of telling your daughter something you know will change her life forever.

Within four hours, I was burying the emotions of this horrific event with food. I had left home without a plan to help me stay compliant with my weight loss while we were away. I wasn't prepared, physically or emotionally.

So the two of us ate together. We cried together. We stuffed down our feelings. We were not equipped with the tools we needed to address this loss any other way. As a result, I gained 8 pounds within 10 days.

You can sympathize and say it was okay because of the trauma we were dealing with. But no—that's just an excuse. This would not be the last life challenge or shock I faced. But because I never wanted to go back to being fat, this was the moment that forced me to identify and develop many of the tools I'm sharing with you here.

You can develop the skills and strength to deal with trauma, even the death of loved ones, while still caring for yourself.

My why was always Sophie. Now my why is to live a long, healthy life so she doesn't feel the pain of losing a parent again anytime soon, and to ensure that when she needs it, she knows exactly how to navigate the pain of loss in a healthy way.

REALITY HITS AGAIN AND AGAIN

After that experience, I committed to developing tools that would help me better navigate life's challenges. I refused to find myself unprepared the next time life took a swing. And it did, less than four months later.

My dad suffered a massive stroke. We had only minutes to decide whether we would opt for brain surgery or let him die. Thankfully, he came through, but he spent more than a month in intensive care and a rehabilitation center. I'm not sure I could have devised a harder test for the tools I developed. But I'm glad to say that they worked.

My response to stress was to stuff my emotions away through eating. I worked extremely hard to ensure I don't do that anymore, but it means navigating through difficult feelings in a new way. It takes practice. I have to dig deep. But I am determined, and there are signs every day that my practice is turning into new habits. I am a work in progress. But when times are challenging, I have to remember that I have already survived lots of difficult times.

My why started when I decided I was done being sick and miserable, and I hated that I taught my daughter the same toxic relationship to food. In addition, people near and dear to me were battling controllable health issues at a young age, and I was scared they were going to die. When Sophie's dad passed, it became clear to me, and I wrote this:

> *"I don't want to leave Sophie without*
> *either of her parents."*

Though Sophie will always be at the core of what drives me to learn more, live better, and never give up, my why also has new inspiration—you. Throughout the process of taking my life back and going from fat to free, I found that I can help others while still taking care of myself. Years of struggles, pain, loss, sadness, and the extraordinary amount of food I ate have afforded me the opportunity to do what I have always enjoyed—making an impact. Every comment I receive, every letter written, and every question asked about how I did this has become a new why.

FREE: AUGUST 22, 2019

I keep telling myself that feeling emotions is so much better than stuffing them away with food. Crying is still uncomfortable for me, and I seem to do it so much more lately. Thank goodness my life is filled with incredible moments right now. It's what fuels me to take new steps each day. Lots of change in my future. I'm scared!

> ### YOUR LESSON:
> *Always come back to your why.*

FAT TO FREE ACTION PLAN

Find your why. Write the full story in your journal. It doesn't have to be pretty; it just has to be true.

Having trouble getting started? Here are some questions you can answer.

◇ What is your motivation to keep going?

◇ Have you hit a rock-bottom moment that inspired you to move?

◇ What reminder will help you keep going when it gets hard?

The truth can be hard to accept, but it's easier when you identify and accept the emotions that are involved.

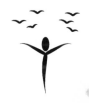

CHAPTER TWO:
MORE THAN
TWO COOKIES

FAT: FEBRUARY 23, 2006

It hurt too much today. I buried the emotions by eating. I know the pain is there, but now I can't feel it.

EMOTIONAL EATING

Emotional eating has become a buzzword among those of us dealing with weight loss. MedicineNet.com defines it as "the practice of consuming large quantities of food—usually 'comfort' or junk foods—in response to feelings instead of hunger." Experts estimate that 75% of overeating is caused by emotions. I'd add to that the addictive qualities of sugar, which is offered up to us in practically everything we consume. Combine those factors with the challenge of needing to consume food so our body works, and it's no wonder so many of us are overweight!

When you research emotional eating, you might see it referred to as stress eating. I always found that to be oversimplified.

Emotional eating can apply to all emotions, regardless of whether they are good or bad. You'll have to decide whether you eat a slice of birthday cake to celebrate, indulge in chocolates on Valentine's Day, or grab a doughnut at a staff meeting. These are all examples of using food for reasons other than simply fueling your body properly. It may feel like too much at this point for you to wrap your mind around breaking those traditions. So for right now, my challenge for you is to simply stay open-minded.

Food is intended as fuel to provide your body with what it needs to function properly. But our society has changed that idea drastically. Throw in the addictive qualities of sugar and it's a recipe for disaster. The cycle of using sustenance for anything other than fuel is strong, addictive, and hard to break when FOOD IS EVERYWHERE!

DO YOU HAVE A TOXIC RELATIONSHIP WITH FOOD?

You have to start by being honest with yourself. Identifying addictive behaviors can help you realize any issues you must address.

Ask yourself these questions:

◇ Do I ever crave a specific food?

◇ Do I keep eating even after a meal is finished?

◇ Do I eat faster than others?

◇ Do I eat immediately after an emotional event, whether I'm happy or sad?

◇ Do I ever experience guilt after eating?

Did you answer yes to any of those? In that case, your food choices likely only deliver temporary relief and result in negative consequences such as added weight, poor health, relationship issues, shame, guilt, and watching life pass you by while you wish it were different. Does that sound like you? If so, you may have an unhealthy relationship with food.

Emotional eating exists on a spectrum. Behaviors may be as simple as thinking you have to clear your plate at every meal, or as shameful as hiding in a parking lot to eat large quantities of food just to distract yourself from hurting. Emotional eating can relate to boredom, fear, awkwardness, anger, excitement, or anticipation. You name the emotion—if you're eating rather than navigating through those feelings, that's emotional eating.

Everyone eats for emotional reasons sometimes. What makes the relationship toxic is *quantity* and *frequency*. Plenty of people eat just one cookie, a small bowl of ice cream, or a few fries. But if you're regularly eating a whole bag of cookies or the entire carton of ice cream, that's another matter entirely.

FAT TO FREE ACTION PLAN

1. Write some examples of what your emotional eating looks like. Make sure it includes the details you are not willing to say out loud. You know, like sneaking more cookies when nobody is looking, digging into your child's candy stash, or eating before you get home only to eat another meal. Or maybe your choices are different and look like snacking while you're putting away leftovers, having dessert when you're not

even hungry, serving up ice cream to celebrate or soothe.

2. Include details about the feelings you have when you're asking yourself, "Why can't I stop?"

3. If you don't know where to start, use the questions above but instead of answering yes or no, provide details such as when you typically do these things and how you are feeling in those moments.

Sharing my story and what I used to do to my body began feeling uncomfortable and filled with guilt, shame, and even some embarrassment but has transformed into testimony that I believe has a purpose and must be shared. The feedback I get from others fuels my desire to shine a light in the shadows and assure people that life doesn't have to be this way.

You can choose to make the change from fat to free. You can take control of food instead of letting it control you. It's astounding how many of us battle the same choices every day. It's time we start talking about it and strive to do better.

WHAT IT LOOKS LIKE

Food used to be on my mind all the time. First thing in the morning, I'd plan what to eat—down in our kitchen, during the drive to work, at work, on the drive home, and for dinner. All day, thoughts of food. I'd be eating a large meal while thinking about my next one. Vacations, weekends, and basically every day was planned around what I'd eat.

Food wasn't only my way of numbing myself, it could also serve as entertainment or even a level of intimacy in my relationships. Everybody needs to eat, so cooking and eating are often times when you can find common ground and bond.

My emotional eating was at its worst when I was a single parent, weighing well over 250 pounds. I was lonely, full of anxiety, and getting worse as I watched every day go by. I lived in a constant state of feeling full. Even a slight tinge of what I thought was hunger and I'd declare that I needed to eat. I ended each night full of food, but still lonely and so sad. I desperately wanted something different.

I have so many journal entries about failed diet and exercise attempts. I worked out—a lot. I was fat but strong. I even won a strength competition at a local gym when I weighed 220 pounds. This was the lowest weight I usually reached before gaining it all back. It was such a vicious cycle. I was slowly killing myself.

Life disappointments, challenges, and hurt kept appearing, and food kept helping me avoid the pain. The fat armor that I believed was protecting me was only harming me. I am an intelligent woman, so deep down I knew. You can see it in my journals. But this knowledge only made it easier to condemn myself through shame and guilt for choosing to perpetuate the cycle and be miserable.

I told myself that if I stayed fat, I'd avoid unwanted attention. But I was lying to myself, because I truly wanted love and companionship. I was desperate for it. I kept eating to avoid feelings and continued to isolate in self-sabotage. The result was a long chain of side effects including anxiety, surgeries, sickness, and eventually Type 2 diabetes. I could not feel my feet. I was on six medications. My kidney doctor told me I was headed for dialysis.

I entered into unhealthy relationships by reasoning, "If they love me despite my weight, I'll know it's true love." The problem with that theory is that my relationships never had a chance because I never brought the real me to the table.

My emotional eating would include eating several days' worth of calories in one meal. Friends and family had no idea. They knew I was fat and unhappy, but they didn't know the extreme toxic relationship I had with food. When you're numbing yourself with food, you find ways to eat while telling yourself that nobody notices. They obviously saw me choosing to eat large quantities for three meals a day, but what they didn't see was what happened between meals. Like when I brought home dinner, I'd order more and eat it in the car before sitting with them, as if I hadn't eaten anything since lunch.

I had several go-to schemes. A big breakfast at home could be followed by a stop at the gas station on the way to work. Depending on my mood, I'd get breakfast sandwiches, a Diet Coke, and sometimes, candy bars or other snacks.

I never hesitated to enjoy treats provided in the office or to help myself to the many desktop chocolate bowls. I enjoyed treating the staff, but my choice to do it with food was selfish, as I needed a pick-me-up when my sugar levels would drop. If my day involved anything stressful, challenging, or even just a schedule change—anything involving a loss of control—I'd hit a drive-thru on the way home. Then I'd sit down to eat a normal dinner with my family. And the cycle would start again the next day.

Why so much food? If you're stuffed to the point that you have to unbutton your pants or need to lie down, it helps you avoid feeling the emotions you're avoiding because you've made yourself so uncomfortable that your mind focuses on that instead. Crying could be stopped in its tracks. Anxiety from feeling out of place can be soothed with baked goods like Costco muffins, cheesecake, or apple pie.

My go-to food was pizza, but it was never just that. It started with Diet Coke, a salad, and wings and was always followed up with something sweet like warm chocolate chip cookies. Much comfort was also found in gas station food (don't judge), including the big hot dogs or a doughy breakfast sandwich, always accompanied with the largest Diet Coke possible. And of course I had to have candy for dessert—even first thing in the morning.

I practiced years of stuffing away any hurt, fear, or emotion. And that led to all those feelings multiplying and getting worse. The more I ate, the fatter I got. My physical pain increased and my emotional pain deepened. It was a dysfunctional cycle of avoidance and pain.

FACING AN ADDICTION

Now I realize that my emotional eating was an addiction. I needed more and more to find the rush, to feel joy. Sugar kept me going back for more. It was a true addiction—a habit, a reaction without thought. What I didn't realize at the time is that acknowledging this addiction would be the key to stopping it.

When my emotional eating was at its worst, it didn't matter if the life challenge was a flat tire, a sick child, or a bad day at work. Food would soothe me, help me avoid the emotions. I felt I was a victim and didn't understand why everybody else had the easy life I wanted. It just didn't seem fair.

News flash: No one has a totally easy life.

But back then, no one could convince me otherwise. Many tried, and I'd see their mouths moving, but in my head, a voice told me, "They just don't understand. They have it so easy." This is a victim mindset at its worst.

When I started this journey, I was filled with regret, sadness, and anger at myself. I started to drop the victim voice and listen to what people had been telling me all along. If I was going to truly heal and become my best self, I needed to love who I was. But it sounded impossible. Years of searching and hearing the answers finally started sinking in. What I believed about how everybody else was living a blessed life with no challenges was not true. What I wished for did not exist.

This is the task that will likely cause you to drag your feet. It's hard. So set it aside for now. We'll come back to it at the end of the book, because I want you to hear a few more messages first.

GETTING STARTED

You might feel too tired to do anything right now. This is a result of the physical challenge of carrying around all of your weight plus the impact of the types and extreme amounts of food you are choosing to put in your body. The kind of tired I'm talking about is when your arms are too exhausted to hold up a hair dryer. Getting ready for the day takes all your energy. And by the time you're dressed, you need a nap.

I blamed my exhaustion on everything but my weight. I fell asleep anywhere, anytime. Did I mention I snored as well? We wrote it off as a family trait. My family always knew that soon after I got into the car, I'd be asleep. Instead of interacting, I was out and sawing logs until we arrived at our destination. I wasn't great company.

And this exhaustion would continue through the entire day. Everything required a lot of effort, so I rarely wanted to participate in activities. In reality, I wanted to do it all and so much more. It was embarrassing when anyone in the family would bring it to my attention.

Are you nodding in agreement? You know it. You live it. You're unable to see beyond it. You're discouraged, and it all feels so heavy. You don't believe that anybody truly understands. You accept it as just who you are. You're the master of avoidance, showing up with a pasted-on smile. You write it off as "not a big deal" even though you know your choices are slowly killing you, physically and emotionally. You've come to accept it.

Even worse, you're causing yourself pain and hurting those around you. You keep it at bay by turning to your only comfort: food. You get through responsibilities, but by the end of the day you're physically exhausted and mentally depressed. By the end of the week, you've given every ounce of energy just to get ready to repeat it all again.

You're crying inside.

You want life to be different.

You want to end your toxic relationship with food.

You need to make a change.

And you absolutely can.

There are two distinct phases of this journey to get you living the life you imagine.

1. You have to learn how to fuel your body.

2. You have to end your toxic relationship with food.

You have many options to choose from, virtually endless information and programs. Code Red was the one that clicked with me, and it was life altering. You need to find yours. Make sure to find one that supports eating real food and cutting out sugar.

Some diets can work (at least for a while), and many have reasonable foundations. You've probably tried diets and even have had some success. But the reason most of these don't work is because you're never getting to the second phase. Diets don't address the core issue of your toxic relationship with food and emotional eating.

We often excuse our own failures because if others are failing too, it must not be possible to lose weight. But it is possible.

You can no longer avoid what you've buried for so long. You must learn to address life and its challenges without turning to food as your comfort, entertainment, or a way to avoid boredom or real feelings.

Buckle up. It's time to change your perspective. Food will no longer serve any purpose in your life other than to fuel your body. Food will no longer be in charge—you will.

FREE: AUGUST 15, 2017

Holy wow! Who knew that you can naturally have this much energy? I had no idea. This morning, I woke up before my alarm and couldn't wait to get out of bed. I don't yawn anymore, and when I get home from work, I'm ready to keep going. Why doesn't anybody tell fat people this stuff? I mean, like pound it into our heads and make us understand that the way we feel is NOT what our bodies are supposed to feel. Who needs Diet Coke when you can feel like this?

> **YOUR LESSON:**
> *Identify your emotional eating as
> it's happening. Call it what it is.*

FAT TO FREE ACTION PLAN

Revisit your why from the last chapter. What did you write in your journal?

1. On a small sheet of paper or index card, narrow your why down to two or three bullet points. They should hit you in the gut when you read them. This reminder is an easy tool that will empower you to think twice before eating your emotions.

2. Now that you can identify the what, where, and when of your emotional eating triggers, make as many copies of that little piece of paper as you need. Tape them all over the house, in your car, and at work to serve as constant reminders. If you prefer an electronic method, you can make it your wallpaper on your phone, iPad, or computer.

The intent of this activity is to become your own coach, your own support system. As you head into the kitchen or you realize there's chocolate in your office or your day starts getting off track or when life gets hard, you'll have a visual cue to bring you back to reality.

The next steps can be difficult as you begin to take full responsibility for your own life. But I know you can do it, and I'll be there every step of the way.

CHAPTER THREE:
IT'S ALL A CHOICE

FAT: DECEMBER 28, 2013

I feel gross! So much junk and not eating well. I'm going to choose differently and start exercising! First class—January 6th. Excited!

April 28, 2014

Trying again. I want to live. Been a difficult couple of months. Lost focus on myself. Good choices today.

May 6, 2014

229 lbs. Difficult pill to swallow, but watch out because I've got a goal. Doing this for me. Good choices for me.

September 19, 2015

Will this be the time I finally choose a different path? Started the Isagenix diet today.

HEARING THE MESSAGE

For years, I heard people simplify all of this, saying it was just a choice to be overweight. I heard it, but I ignored it because I believed nobody could possibly understand how my life was so much harder than theirs. I had convinced myself that the life challenges I experienced were different somehow and I couldn't choose my way out of them.

The truth is, everyone I thought had it so much easier simply knew that their lives were their responsibility. They understood the power of mindset, and they had the skills and information you're learning now.

As I've said before, everybody has a hard life in some way. Everybody also has a choice about how they respond. That's the absolute "secret" to this journey. You might think you've been given the short end of the stick. But everything you do comes down to making different choices than you have in the past. Accepting your responsibility is the mindset change necessary for you to have the life you want.

Not ready to hear that? It's okay. Like I said, I heard it for years (as shown in my journal entries above), but it wasn't until I was honestly ready that the message finally got through.

I remember the exact moment it hit me, right in the middle of my heart. At the same time, my mind shifted.

My company was experiencing a public nightmare, and I was thrust into a spotlight, where I wasn't comfortable. We had learned months earlier that Sophie's dad was an alcoholic, and he eventually landed in the ICU. Then my brother Ted had seven strokes within a week and was also in ICU. My 10-year relationship was struggling, and I was feeling extremely alone.

Because life was hard, I was eating like I usually did, getting fatter and unhealthier. While I was overwhelmed with caring for everyone around me, my doctor started to prepare me for insulin. My eyesight got worse, and I could hardly feel my toes. Every time I felt a new sensation, ache, or pain, I wondered what was failing. I would end each day terrified that my life was getting shorter and that I might not wake up in the morning.

One day, I was chatting with Ted in the ICU. I was on one of my usual rants about our bad genes making us fat. I had watched my mom battle her weight all her life. Same with me and my brothers. My dad was skin and bones, but he also ate a ton of terrible food. As Ted lay flat on his back in the hospital listening to my usual excuses, he suddenly sat up, looked me right in the eyes, and said, "No, Elizabeth! It's a choice!"

I physically felt his words, and it finally made sense. It was like a smack on my forehead, an electrical shock through my body. I filled with a warmth and energy that was different than any time before. In that exact moment, I knew that I was going to change my life.

YOUR RESPONSIBILITY

This may be hard to hear and might even make you angry, but if you accept that your life is your choice, you also have to accept that what your life has been up to this point has also been your choice. That can be a hard pill to swallow.

You might just not be ready to hear this yet, and that's okay. It takes time. It's also another choice you have to own. Just keep reading, because there will be plenty of aha moments to lead you to action, and the day will come when you realize you're in charge of your life.

You might be thinking, *But wait, Elizabeth...*

...I didn't choose for my loved one to die.

...I didn't choose to be a victim of sexual assault.

...I didn't choose for my marriage to end.

And you're absolutely correct. But life challenges, big and small, will always happen. And you have 100% control over how you'll respond. It's your choice whether to stay in a victim role.

This mindset shift will result in powerful and joyful changes. Life is never going to stop challenging you, but with practice, you will gain the strength to respond differently—without involving food.

When I walked out of Ted's hospital room, I started choosing my life, and I was pretty sure I was going to do it through weight-loss surgery. I was done being fat and was finally taking charge.

CHOOSE YOU

The decision was made. I was going to change my life once and for all and get these 100 extra pounds off my body. I declared it. I owned it. I knew enough about weight-loss surgery to know that afterward you had to drink your meals for a while, then eat like a bird.

But I still had a major problem: How on earth could I keep that up when every time I felt any kind of emotion, I ran for fast food? So I hatched a second plan. I'd schedule the surgery but, in the meantime, I'd sign up for a weight-loss challenge. The challenge lasted 45 days. If I couldn't maintain control of my eating for that long, I had no business having a portion of my stomach removed or a band inserted to make it smaller. It would be a death sentence.

I scheduled an orientation for the weight-loss surgery and explained my plan to the surgeon. He laughed at me.

He said, "I'm afraid you won't be successful in the program. In fact, I need you to gain *more* weight to get your BMI up higher so insurance will pay for the surgery."

I was pissed! I stomped out of his office, threw away all the documents, and knew I'd never be back. He had saved my life, but not in the way I had anticipated.

I was done with excuses. I recognized that refusing to spend time working on my thoughts and mindset was just another excuse. I started some research, which eventually led me here to share this advice with you.

Ending your toxic relationship with food will take hard work in many areas of your life, but if you take it one step at a time, you can absolutely do it.

CHOOSE HARD

My brother John helped me realize how strong I was. I was facing the end of a 10-year relationship and moving out. I'd be a single empty nester at the age of 49. This meant big change. It meant being alone. My emotions were off the charts. Eating through it was no longer an option, so I had to feel it all.

I shared these feelings with my tribe, those who love and accept me no matter what. John said he wasn't concerned and he knew I'd be just fine. He pointed out how I had survived a divorce and Sophie being born underweight. He reminded me how I had gone back to college and thrived in my career, all while I was a single parent. How I had dealt with Sophie's dad being an alcoholic and eventually dying from his disease. John helped me realize that my perspective and judgment of myself had been so different than others. I had only focused on what I deemed as failures.

I made it through it all. I gave my heart and so much more to so many. Now I know that I can do anything. I'm not sure that John even knows the impact that his love for me made at that moment.

Thoughts result in action and are the first steps to everything. "Approximately 40% of our thoughts each day are actually habits." (Haden, 2020) Nearly half! In effect, we are just all mindlessly walking through our days, running on autopilot.

Don't settle for that. Set your standards high. You have control over your thoughts and your actions. Some of them may work out and some won't. But the great thing is that you have 100% control over how you respond when things don't work out.

You also have 100% control over what food you put in your mouth. It's your choice. Every time. It starts with a thought. It becomes an action. It's a choice. You can choose your life to be what you want it to be.

FREE: OCTOBER 22, 2017

My future self: I have learned to feel and embrace the emotions rather than stuff them,

I am true to myself, I let go of the past and am now surrounded by a tribe who lifts me up, I am healthy and confident and enjoy experiences in life rather than food, and I share my journey to help inspire others to bring their true selves to the table. I love myself.

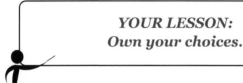

YOUR LESSON:
Own your choices.

FAT TO FREE ACTION PLAN

Work on a few thoughts each day to help shift your mindset into a strong foundation. Those will inform the actions you must take to reach your goals.

When you decide to change your mindset, here are some ways you can break it down into manageable, actionable steps.

◇ Focus on the good, no matter how small it may be. Find the blessings in everything that happens. If you're stuck, just be thankful you woke up and have air in your lungs that day. Many find it helpful to write out three blessings at the end of their day.

◇ Find humor in bad or difficult moments. Laughter helps! It causes the release of endorphins, which promotes well-being and can even relieve pain. It can also lower blood pressure and reduce stress hormones.

◇ Live in the moment. Depression is often associated with living in the past, and anxiety is associated with living in the future. The only reality is right now. You can't change the past and you can't control the future. Be present.

◇ Switch negative self-talk to positive. This includes any time you slide into an old mindset. It will happen, so simply acknowledge it, then make the choice to move on.

◇ Surround yourself with positive-minded people.

◇ Start viewing your mistakes as lessons. Practice will make you even better equipped to handle difficult situations in the future. Write about what happened. Maybe you snapped at your kids or a coworker. Rewrite it to detail the valuable lessons you learned and how grateful you are for that opportunity. Then create a plan for handling similar situations better in the future.

For example:

◇ I snapped at my kids for spilling milk.

◇ I am grateful that I realized my response was inappropriate.

◇ This will be a great opportunity to share with my kids about how everyone makes mistakes, but as long as you apologize and do better next time, that's how we learn and grow.

◇ Next time they make a mess, I will take a deep breath and say to myself, "Oh brother." Then I will smile and think of my kid's feelings first.

◇ "Uh-oh, how can we clean up this mess?"

Another example would be snacking in the evening.

◇ I chose to snack last night.

◇ I am grateful that I realized that is not a choice in line with my goals.

◇ This is a great opportunity to address my eating out of boredom rather than the need to fuel my body, and next time I will be prepared with safeguards to make different choices.

◇ Next time I feel the desire to snack in the evening, I will pull out my list of other activities I can do instead and lean on my tribe to help me change my course.

These are all habits you can build. They do take time and practice, but for now, draw strength knowing that you're taking a first step to changing your mindset and ending your toxic relationship with food. You are getting off the sidelines.

CHAPTER FOUR:
I'LL BE HAPPY
WHEN I'M SKINNY

FAT: DECEMBER 7, 2015

My life in five years: I will be a healthy, active 50-year-old who weighs no more than 150 lbs. I will be confident in my body and willing to try new things. My finances will be strong and allow me to do activities I am scared of doing, including travel. My life will be active, including family activities like riding bikes, hiking, and vacations.

If I don't accomplish these goals, I will die. If I don't accomplish these goals, I will have failed in teaching Sophie that her body and health are priorities. If I don't accomplish these goals, I will continue to miss out on life and hide from my fears by sitting at home. If I don't accomplish these goals, I will always wonder what it would feel like to be healthy.

OPA!

Sixth grade was one of my first memories of trying to fit in, always feeling excluded, and working hard to be considered a "cool kid." It was also the first point in my life I remember my mom responding to challenges by trying to fix them rather than letting me figure out how to navigate on my own. We still lived in Georgia. Streetlights were our clocks, hoses were our water fountains, and you knew where everyone was hanging out by the number of bikes on the front lawn.

That year, I auditioned for a school play and didn't get a part. I was heartbroken. I went home and shared my disappointment with my mom. Her fixing instincts kicked in, and the sting of rejection was calmed with some of her best comfort foods. Then she called my teacher and asked to meet.

I appreciate that my mom's response was always to love me and try to help me feel better. But I missed many opportunities to feel rejection. Even worse, the teacher's solution was to add a new part to the show. Now I had one line at the end: "Opa!" (Opa is simply an exclamation of excitement, like saying "Woo-hoo!") The absurdity of the line and obvious coddling only led to giggles from my classmates. I don't even remember what the play was about, but the feelings of embarrassment lasted for years.

I was always working to change or conform to what I interpreted as cool. I was in search of the coolest jeans, party invitations, and roller-skating dates. I desperately wanted to be included. After the school play fiasco, I knew exactly what I needed to do. I was going to get some new clothes and style my hair just like the most popular girl, Jennifer. She had full, thick hair that came down to her shoulders and had the most perfect feathering.

Ever supportive, my mom took me shopping and to the salon just in time for class pictures. Walking into school with my new three-piece outfit (a skirt, blouse, and blazer) along with my incredibly hip new hairstyle was going to make everyone want to be my friend. And then I'd feel happy and accepted.

But because I was in the sixth grade, I failed to realize two points:

1. Finding happiness and acceptance from a new look is incredibly unrealistic.

2. If you took my hair and tried to mimic that style, you ended up with a disaster instead!

I walked into that school with my head held high. But in reality, the feathering had left me with one solid curl down each side of my face. It looked like I had wrapped my hair around a curling iron and then failed to brush it afterward. I will never forget the laughter. My classmates had smirks and snide comments the minute I walked into that classroom.

Instantly, my expectations of greatness circled the drain and tears filled my eyes. I was so confused. What I didn't understand that day was that my expectations had been unrealistic from the beginning. I wasn't addressing what I should have.

SITTING ON THE SIDELINES

Are you on sitting the sidelines of your life, convinced that when you lose weight everything will be better? Just as winning the lottery won't make you happy, neither will a number on the scale. You need to change your expectations. Weight loss doesn't equal self-respect that you never had in the first place.

Setting appropriate expectations is critical; otherwise, you'll reach your goal weight and find that you still turn to food to avoid uncomfortable feelings, relieve boredom, or be entertained. Weight loss doesn't make you happy, fix relationships, or end your toxic relationship with food any more than buying different clothes and changing your hair makes you feel accepted and loved.

When I was deciding whether to have weight-loss surgery, I had to be sure I could change my relationship with food first. I had to adjust any expectation that surgery would be a quick fix and that hopefully I could face the rest of it later.

You can eat less and exercise. You can have surgery, drink shakes, take pills, and eat grapefruit all day, and it might change a number on the scale, but if you're expecting that to solve all your other challenges, you're always going to end up back at square one.

It's time to break the cycle! Adjust your expectations. Weight loss will improve your health and overall per-formance. The number on the scale will go down. You'll have more energy, you'll be able to wear smaller clothes, you might feel some increased confidence, and will likely enjoy many other wonderful benefits.

But when you change your mindset to health instead of just a lower weight, when you change your thoughts and take action to end your toxic relationship with food, you will have much greater control over it. Along the way, you'll develop new habits, face your fears, and begin responding to life's challenges without food. You'll finally accept that you're 100% in control of your life. And you'll realize that loving yourself is not selfish.

The greatest advantage of these choices is the example I had started to set for my loved ones. They didn't believe I could stick with it and change, and frankly I didn't blame them. Sophie had been watching my struggles for 17 years and she was certainly following in my footsteps. I was determined to show her that things could be different.

She actually joined me in my efforts and ended up losing 40 pounds! The day I dropped her off at college, I knew that I had given her the tools she needed to take care of herself and fuel her body properly. I am a proud mom knowing that she has figured out how to do that all while living in the dorms at college.

RESET YOUR EXPECTATIONS

This is not a quick fix. It will be a forever-evolving journey as you learn and grow. You won't just cross a finish line, pat yourself on the back, and say you're off to the next project. Commitment to go from fat to free requires the understanding that you're choosing a healthy lifestyle, and it requires effort every single day. But what you'll learn through this process will undoubtedly lead you to look at other aspects of your life where you can apply your new skills as well.

I recommend you figure out what actions you'll take to fuel your body, then take action. If your end goal is to be healthy and end your toxic relationship with food, you must know how to properly fuel your body. Neither step works without the other. If you don't fuel your body the way it was intended, you can put an end to your addiction to food but still be fat.

FAT TO FREE ACTION PLAN

Research how you want to fuel your body. Dive in. Do not do it half-assed. Remember this step is key to this process. Keep your eye out for gimmicks that want you to buy their foods. The key you should be looking for in any plan is that it allows you to fuel your body with real food.

You should be aware that when you stop eating all the bad food, you'll likely feel crappy at first. You might have a headache, muscle aches, extreme exhaustion, or a feeling of being run-down. But this is actually a good first step, because your body needs to detox from the unhealthy foods you used to eat. And you'll find increased energy and excitement from seeing the scale go down, which will inspire you to keep pushing forward. After a week or two, your moods will stabilize, which will be helpful as you start feeling emotions more intensely without food as a crutch.

Your journey will be filled with unexpected events. Some are going to challenge you, and some are going to give you more joy than you ever imagined. The challenges may be something like noticing all the negatives in your life, loved ones not being supportive, or changes in relationships with friends.

The joy will be having energy unlike you have experienced before, your body not aching, decreasing medications, increased confidence, wearing new clothes, having your weight match your driver's license, fitting in small chairs, not needing a seat-belt extender on the airplane, riding a bike again, playing with your kids, or being able to wear your wedding ring again.

I could write a whole book just about the joy you will experience. Embracing the journey and letting go of any associated fear takes out any emotional charge you attached to it. You always have control over your responses, your actions, and the meaning and importance you assign to moments in your life.

FREE: SEPTEMBER 10, 2019

Holy crap, it's quiet in this house. This "facing your fears" stuff is for the birds. I don't like being alone. I keep hearing that pesky voice in my head about how it will be good for me and it will help me learn more about myself. But that doesn't make me feel better.

Single and an empty nester is not what I had in mind for this year. I miss Sophie. I miss my bonus kids. [Sophie was off in college and my relationship ended so I no longer lived with my bonus kids.] I must pull myself together. Practice what I preach. Be thankful.

I was able to park in the garage and squeeze out of a tiny parking space. Okay, that was pretty dang cool. Tomorrow is a new day.

> *YOUR LESSON:*
> *Have realistic expectations.*

FAT TO FREE ACTION PLAN

Write one sentence outlining your weight and non-weight goals. Be specific.

For example...

"I want to weigh 140 pounds, take no medications, and be active at least three times a week."

Sit back and visualize what you want to accomplish and what your life will look like. Then keep reading to learn how to break this down into smaller goals and objectives.

CHAPTER FIVE:
IT'S NOT YOUR FAULT

FAT: JUNE 10, 2007

What is it with me? I'm weepy and I can't stop thinking about what I don't have. Is Jamie right? Am I a victim? Do I want to stay alone? What could I be doing different right at this minute that would directly impact my being alone, being happy?

August 11, 2013

I'm not sure how to do all that I need. I'm scared. I feel alone. My foot hurts bad. I'm scared I'm going to die.

A SAD CYCLE

My foot hurt because my diabetes was out of control. I could barely feel my toes anymore. By this time, I had broken that same foot twice—once requiring surgery. My body was slowly deteriorating.

This kind of journal entry was common. So was crying in the shower and carrying around a constant feeling of disappointment. Excuses were endless. My victim mentality was strong. Those who tried to help just didn't understand—well that's what I told them, and myself, anyway. I felt defeated and believed life would never change.

Most days, I showed up to obligations with a smile on my face, determined to mask my anxiety, pain, and sadness from everyone. I worked hard to be the happy, fat girl with tons of energy. But I don't think I fooled anyone, not even myself.

I spent weekends recovering on the couch, eating takeout, sleeping, and keeping the guilt at bay by getting up every couple of hours to run a load of laundry or do the dishes. I felt accomplished at the end of a weekend if I had gotten routine chores done. Then I got up Monday morning and did it all again. The soundtrack to this sad, steady cycle were arguments and bickering about going out to have fun versus staying home. Exhaustion, shame, and disappointment won those arguments damn near every time, which means nobody won at all.

You would think I was sitting here consumed by regret as I share these stories. And I'm not going to lie—there is some. However, if I hadn't lived the life I did, I wouldn't be here today sharing my journey to help others.

And I know there are many people who feel trapped in this sad cycle. I see you. I see it in your walk. I see it in your exhaustion. I hear it when you're talking to your children. I want to help you.

You see, I had convinced myself that all the pain and sadness weren't my fault. I was sure I had been chosen to endure a harder life than anyone else. Life always seemed to pile on top of me. I didn't understand why so many others lived with what seemed like great ease and blessings.

Many hours of counseling, reading self-help books, and attending conferences finally led me to realize I was living a victim life. I learned to play a victim early. I don't remember how long I had been doing it, but when you realize you can get more attention after something negative happens, it starts to become a behavior. This was ingrained at an early age, and I continued to use it as a coping strategy.

One time during a counseling session, my therapist said, "Elizabeth, this..." He held his hand above his head. "This up here—this level of life you think others are living—just doesn't exist. We all have to face different struggles. Your response to is to live and dwell on those struggles and get what you need from the negativity. That's being a victim."

I learned that I was missing the knowledge and skill to respond to life's challenges in a positive manner. Everyone I assumed had it so easy just knew how to handle challenges instead of dwelling on them. It's not that life was easier for them; they just didn't let every setback completely tell the story of their lives.

◊ Are you living with a victim mentality?

◊ Do you resent whenever your life is not the way you want it to be but fail to take any ownership of that being your choice?

◊ Do you focus on everyone else's life rather than living your own?

◊ Are you always working to meet the needs of others out of fear of ending up alone?

◊ Is everyone else a priority over your own needs, out of a sense of martyrdom or self-sacrifice?

TIME TO ACT

Okay, tough love time. This section might seem a little harsh, but it's something you need to hear to finally shake yourself awake and make this critical change. Please know that it's written with much love for you and the confidence that you'll succeed.

Recognizing that you're living a victim life may look like ending all of the excuses for why you cannot make the choices you should in order to lose weight or accomplish other goals. You believe that anything bad that happens in your life is not your fault, and nobody understands because your life is more difficult than others. Your tire went flat. A key meeting was canceled. You were not asked to join your friends to go out. You spilled food in the kitchen. Your furnace broke. You have an excuse for everything. You're stuck believing the world is against you.

Guess what? That's all just part of life. Why do you keep eating the shit sandwich and expecting it to taste different?

But you can stop right now. Choose it!

Stop blaming others. This is just another form of making excuses. It's not an effective way to achieve your goals and will keep you stuck. Take ownership of your life. Turn the finger around and point it at yourself. In any given situation, ask yourself what your role was.

You'll never be able to control what someone else did to you, but you can 100% control your reaction. Maybe you got stood up for a date, a loved one insulted you, a child said something mean, a coworker got the promotion over you. Regardless of what happened in those scenarios, the only control you have is your reaction. Don't be a victim.

Stop self-loathing. What led you to believe that you're not worth the same love and care you provide for so many others? Did you make a bad decision in the past and convince yourself it was unforgivable and that you're not worthy?

I have news for you: You're not only going to have to love yourself as you are now, you must also learn to love who you were and who you are becoming.

Forgive and move on. What are you holding on to and how is it serving you? Most likely, it's preventing you from moving forward and focusing on your goals. Forgiveness is all about you, not about receiving an apology. It's a *choice* you get to make in response to something that happened to you. If you don't let go of situations you need to forgive, you'll continue to carry negative feelings and let them impact future relationships and events. Holding on to the past is preventing you from being present and experiencing all you could be learning. Let it go!

You'll recognize that you're no longer living a victim life when you respond to challenges with determination rather than using them as excuses or reasons not to accomplish your goals. You'll push through hard times rather than letting them stop you. When your friends are successful, you'll celebrate with them and not be jealous. Even at times of loss, you'll be able to focus on past joys and memories. Your life will be embraced, and you'll choose to celebrate it and all of its challenges, no matter how hard.

FAT TO FREE ACTION PLAN

Take a few minutes and write out any feelings you experience after reading that you need to take ownership of your life. Be completely honest with yourself. There are no wrong answers here.

FINDING HOPE

During all the years I was overweight, one thing remained constant: hope. At times, it faded to the smallest spark in my eye or feeling in my heart, but it never left.

My job was a blessing for many reasons, but one of the greatest gifts was exposure to good people. I heard numerous stories of others dealing with challenges far exceeding anything I could even imagine, and doing so honorably. My motivation came from them, my daughter, and my family. I kept going, believing something would change. I just didn't know what.

I always believed that my life was meant to be more; when I stopped acting like a victim, it turned out I was right.

IN CASE OF EMERGENCY

Though hope was important, so was being prepared. Life happens without any warning, but there are safeguards you can have in place to help you be successful.

Even the best plans can go by the wayside without any notice. Becoming "hangry" opens the door for bad choices, so pack an emergency body-fueling kit to keep in your car and another one for work. In an emergency, you're in response mode, caretaker mode, and worrying about others instead of how you're going to take care of yourself.

And don't skip this step because your family is close to home or your work doesn't require travel. You never know what might happen, so it's better to be prepared. If you need to travel on short notice, it's great to have a packing checklist and a plan already put together.

FREE: OCTOBER 14, 2019

It's so odd to me still that I can now go on a weekend trip filled with laughter and good friends, playing cards, and shopping, and come home without anxiety to clean the house and get ready for the week. Still uncomfortable, but I'm much closer to living the life I imagined.

> **YOUR LESSON:**
> **Stop being a victim.**

FAT TO FREE ACTION PLAN

You did a lot of emotional work and self-reflection in this chapter. Your "take action" directive is a little different. It's time to make your in-case-of-emergency plan. Life is going to keep challenging and pushing you. But you're not going to be a victim anymore. You're going to be prepared.

Following are some quick reference lists to use when you find yourself in a situation you can't control. Tailor them to your needs so you can respond in the moment without much thought.

Emergency Fuel: Always keep an emergency food reserve with you. This bag, box, or container is specifically for situations that are likely to keep you from eating outside your plan. Your emergency bag should include nonperishable foods to provide you with fuel and carry you through until your next meal. Some suggestions include:

◇ Beef jerky

◇ Canned tuna

◇ Mayo packets

◇ Nuts

◇ Water

Packing: This checklist is also helpful for non-emergency traveling. Your list should apply to your needs, but here are some ideas from mine.

◇ Book

◇ Emergency food bag

◇ Food scale

◇ Gallon jug and water bottle

◇ Headphones

◇ Journal

◇ Measuring spoons

◇ Sleep necessities: eye mask, sleep aid, downloaded meditation recording

◇ Sneakers

◇ Travel bathroom scale

◇ Travel grocery list

A note about your travel grocery list: Out of habit, you might have previously defaulted to eating out or ordering room service when you traveled. Most places you visit likely have nearby grocery stores. Healthy foods you should eat while staying in a hotel include the following:

◇ Cream cheese

◇ Guacamole

◇ Heavy whipping cream for hotel coffee

◇ Pepperoni

◇ Precooked bacon or sausage

◇ Turkey slices

◇ Veggies and ranch dressing

If possible, bring a few plates and utensils. If not, grab some from the hotel lobby or buy them at the store. Plan it all so there is no room for excuses.

Next, outline the actions necessary for you to be successful when away from home. Here are some planning suggestions:

1. Pack an emergency food bag.

2. Ensure your hotel room has a fridge and microwave.

3. Grocery shop no more than 12 hours after arrival.

4. Plan your food intake daily before leaving your hotel room.

5. Continue to weigh in daily.

6. Make time for self-care, like meditating each morning, going to the hotel gym, or taking a stroll around your destination city.

7. Increase your water intake. Traveling is difficult on your body, especially on planes, and can decrease your energy levels. Proper hydration can help avoid fatigue.

8. Share your weight-loss journey with others, and talk about what you'll be doing to stay on track while away from home.

You did not gain this weight overnight, so do not expect it to come off quickly. Your expectations need to be in line with your efforts.

CHAPTER SIX:
SETTING HEALTH GOALS

FAT: DECEMBER 7, 2015

I will print menu plans every Friday. I will plan and shop every Saturday. I will prep cook every Sunday. I will choose home cooking even if it means late dinners. I will get up and prepare my lunches for work every morning. I will try new foods. I will go on no less than a 30-minute walk every weekend.

GOALS AND OBJECTIVES

I didn't lose 100 pounds. Not all at once anyway. It was more like a loss...a gain...a stall...another loss. I just didn't lose 100 pounds all at once. One day at a time. Just as with any major goal in my life.

The journal entry above (or something relatively close to it) is written in many different ways throughout all my years of documenting being fat. It was always the same pattern: set goals, try to reach them, fail, return to my old ways, and repeat. The only change from cycle to cycle was which new gimmick I tried. I always wanted to believe that the next new trend was going to be "the one."

Now I realize that many factors contributed to the cycle I repeated for more than 30 years. For one, I don't think I ever believed that losing 100 pounds was attainable until I was more than halfway there. Confidence is hard to come by when you're as heavy as I was. It's nearly impossible to believe you're suddenly going to be successful after all of those years of trying and failing.

No matter how much weight you want to lose, the task at hand can feel beyond your reach, and that opens the gates for self-doubt. You've probably tried time and again only to end up back at the beginning. The problems come if you continue to expect success even though you're not actually taking action.

Most likely, the suggestions that follow aren't going to be new to you. But while you likely apply these techniques in other areas of your life, you may not have considered applying them to weight loss.

⬦ Break each goal down into smaller tasks. You can work on one or two each day, which ultimately leads you to task completion over time. This makes your weight-loss goals manageable.

The more success you have, the more energized you'll be to work on these small objectives. The progress will inspire you to stay focused and committed. This is a marathon, not a sprint. Your goal is to behave differently so you'll succeed where you've failed so many times in the past. Don't expect perfection—you're in this for the long haul.

⬦ Develop a method to track your success. Your goal should be to lose weight each day, and your objectives to support that goal should be measurable.

For example:

- ◆ I will get no less than seven hours of sleep every night.

- ◆ I will drink a gallon of water each day.

- ◆ I will not reward my efforts, replace boredom, or numb feelings by eating.

◇ Establish a system of measurement that's appealing to you. It helps to have a visual you can glance at to know when you're making strides. You'll want little pats on the back as you go.

Now I'm not crafty or creative, so I simply posted my weight log on the bathroom mirror. Each morning, I'd log my weight. I circled every Friday because that was the day I'd step back and analyze how I was doing. I didn't allow myself to stress during the week if I didn't lose as much as I had hoped, or if I gained weight. Each sheet had 30 days and separate goals.

I kept all of them because I still find it helpful to go back and look at the hard work I did each day and how it added up over time.

If you'd like to get more creative, you could create an elaborate board and represent every pound with a colorful sticky note. Or use two jars: one empty and one filled with marbles to represent your current pounds. As you lose a pound, move a marble from one jar to the next. Get creative!

◇ Set aside 10 minutes every night to review your day and prepare for the next one.

◇ Dedicate at least 30 minutes each week to review your goals and daily objectives. Identify where you're having success and where you may need to adjust. Choose to make this time a priority.

REWARDING SUCCESS

Just as important as setting goals and objectives is finding new non-food rewards. What is rewarded is repeated. Reward yourself in order to draw out positive emotions and create a new cycle. Meeting your objectives and putting in the effort results in positive rewards. Likely you used to do this with food, which would trigger a dopamine response and light up the reward circuitry in your brain. So now you must find a way to trigger the response through non-food rewards.

Ensure the goals you set require some effort so you feel deserving of the rewards. They should be appropriate for the level of work and happen as soon as you meet the goal. They don't have to be lavish or extravagant. Rewards should be physically and emotionally healthy and make you feel joy.

I highly recommend experiences you've always wanted to try. Activities like bike riding, taking a walk, or hiking are great rewards. Have you ever ordered flowers for yourself? Maybe just sleeping in late one day would feel like a reward. One suggestion a client shared with me is aromatherapy. She liked to reward herself by putting on her favorite lotion or lighting a scented candle. All of these events can ignite joy.

> *Tip: Wear teeth-whitening strips while you're preparing food so you're not tempted to nibble!*

FAT TO FREE ACTION PLAN

1. Make a list of rewards to reference when you have a small success. This will save you time so you can simply pick from the list instead of trying to figure out what you want in the moment.

2. Make a second list of rewards for when you accomplish your goals. Remember, they should match the work you did. For example, in my opinion, losing 50 pounds would match treating yourself to a spa day.

You should also practice a rewards system with your family, especially if you have kids. The most common response to children when they have done something good is to offer ice cream or candy or to take them out to eat. Instead, give them the gift of your time. Kids rarely care what you do—just give them your undivided attention. Play cards, read a book, watch a movie, go on a bike ride, or color a picture together.

Ask your family to help develop a reward list and post it on the refrigerator. When they have done something deserving, they can pick an activity from the list. Break the cycle of food as reward, and arm your children with new incentives to set and reach their goals.

Here are some ideas of ways you could reward yourself.

◇ Go for a walk.

◇ Journal.

◇ Color.

◇ Listen to music.

◇ Dance.

◇ Exercise.

◇ Call a friend.

◇ Get a massage.

◇ Rent a movie.

What brings you joy? By writing this out, you can look at the list and pick one. No thinking required. It's going to take all your strength to keep food out of your mouth. If one activity doesn't work, try the next.

Ask your friends and family to help you build this list. Your support system will be a big part of your commitment to non-food rewards.

FREE: AUGUST 8, 2019

One baby step at a time. I'm looking around, a bit off guard about where I am today. I did this? I lost 100 lbs. and have been keeping it off. I realize it more when I see the looks on the faces of others. They are genuinely shocked. And as of today, I'm going to start helping others do the same.

I feel a bit like I am free-falling. Not feeling tons of confidence that I'm going to land on my feet. The odd part is that I keep going. I think I finally get that I am in control. I control the steps I take and at what pace. Staying in the moment makes it a bit easier to keep going.

> **YOUR LESSON:**
> **Set goals and objectives. Find appropriate rewards.**

FAT TO FREE ACTION PLAN

1. Revisit the goal you wrote in Chapter Four.

2. Break it down into objectives.

3. Devise a plan for how and when you will accomplish them.

4. Decide how you will reward yourself once the goal is met.

For example:

◊ **Goal:** I want to lose 50 pounds in the next 10 months.

◊ **Objective:** I will lose 10 pounds this month.

◊ **Plan**

   ♦ I will not snack in the evenings.

   ♦ I will read at least one article or listen to one podcast per day teaching me how to change my habits.

   ♦ I will follow all the rules of the weight-loss plan I have chosen to assist me in weight loss.

◊ **Reward:** After losing 10 pounds this month, I will reward myself with a 30-minute bath that does not involve a phone, pets, or children anywhere around!

You know why you are doing this, you know what it is, and you have some goals. Now it's time to examine your relationship with food a bit more closely.

CHAPTER SEVEN:
ARE YOU HUNGRY?

FAT: AUGUST 17, 2013

Two weeks of eating differently. Not much change. Frustrated. Going to log everything. See who can review it and help.

8:00 a.m.: 4 pieces of bacon, 2 slices of sharp cheese

1:30 p.m.: hamburger patty, small piece of steak, A.1. sauce

2:30 p.m.: 6 almonds

4:30 p.m.: I cup of Caesar salad and ½ piece of cheese pizza (first bread in 16 days)

7:00 p.m.: 6 chicken legs cooked in butter, hot wing sauce, carrots, celery, and ranch dip

FOOD IS EVERYWHERE

Yes, you read that right: six chicken legs. I have days, months, and years of logs just like that. Some even worse. I didn't understand why my blood sugar was off the charts and my weight was all over the place. I still get angry at some people in the medical community because they assured me that if I just ate six small meals a day and worked out, the weight would come off. Meanwhile, any medical issues would be treated with pills or surgery.

But with that combination, I would have died at an early age.

Failure and shame continued to mount. I was a food addict who used it to soothe, entertain, or avoid. When would it stop? Food was everywhere.

I never allowed myself to feel hungry, because hungry meant out of control, and that was a trigger for me. I lived in a constant state of fullness. Loss of control was a particularly uncomfortable feeling for me, so whenever I felt it, I'd start shoving enough food in my mouth so I could feel overly full instead. Disgustingly full.

In reality, it wasn't better, just different. If I felt like crying, stuffing myself with food would physically stop that from happening. To me, this meant I had control. But the relief was temporary, and the damage was far worse than if I had just cried.

Crying is okay! Somehow I learned that I should never cry and that asking for help was a sign of weakness. I have memories of my brothers announcing, "She's crying again."

You must prepare for the overwhelming amount of emotions that will arrive once you stop stuffing them down with food. They will leave you feeling uncomfortable. So cry. Cry again. Cry some more. Scream if you want. Feel it. Let it out. Crying has somehow been connected to weakness, but that's just ridiculous.

You're sensitive, compassionate, caring, and aware. Embrace it.

You might even notice—as I did when I'd let go and have a good cry followed by a good night's sleep—that your weight will drop. There's a lot to be said for releasing stress.

ARE YOU HUNGRY?

Are you hungry? Are you sure? How do you know? What does it feel like?

Identifying emotional cues versus hunger cues is vital to your weight-loss success. It's time to start listening to your body. You have to become familiar with your emotions and body responses. This may be out of your comfort zone because it means you stop putting all your energy into others and start investing in yourself.

Hunger cues are easier to identify since they are physical responses from your body. But if you haven't experienced them in a long time, you'll need to learn to listen to your body. It will let you know. You may hear your stomach growling, gurgling, or rumbling. You may have a feeling of emptiness, maybe even a headache, lack of concentration, or nausea.

This part was challenging for me, because to discover what being hungry felt like, I had to give up my habit of comforting with food and realize I was okay. At different times between meals, sit alone, observe what your body is doing, and realize that you're okay. You're in control and nothing bad is happening while you feel the hunger responses.

In fact, when you learn to fuel your body properly, you'll realize that being empty is healthy and gives your body a chance to reset. Our bodies are not meant to be stuffed with processed food all the time.

ARE YOU FULL?

Another essential aspect of learning to listen to your body is identifying when you're full. How do you know when to put the fork down? Stuffing yourself to feel full is likely a habit every time you eat. Your new habit is to eat until you're no longer hungry. There's a big difference. You should not feel heavy, weighed down, sick, nauseated, or numb after eating.

Be mindful of what is on your plate and how much your body truly needs to function properly. This is part of ending your toxic relationship with food. Food is fuel and nothing more.

You may experience some grief around accepting this change. You're ending a long-standing relationship with food. It might seem odd to refer to it as a "relationship," but consider all your memories centered around food. You can absolutely mourn it as a loss. You're letting go of a security blanket in your life that has allowed you to navigate through difficult situations. Food has been a part of family celebrations, social events, times of joy, and moments of grief.

When you think about eating, ask yourself whether it's because you're truly hungry or for another reason.

◊ Are you bored?

◊ Are you eating because you always do at this time of day, or maybe while you're watching TV?

◊ Are you upset or annoyed?

◇ Did something stressful just happen at work?

◇ Did your children upset you?

◇ Are you tired but can't go to bed?

◇ Are you worrying about something?

◇ Is your spouse or loved one upset with you?

◇ Did you just learn you need a new roof on the house?

◇ Are you dealing with financial struggles?

◇ Are you sick?

◇ Are you celebrating something or someone?

◇ Are you preparing food so just one nibble won't hurt?

◇ Did you just walk by the kitchen and see the cookies so you grabbed one?

◇ Did someone give you food and insist that you try a bite?

◇ Are you eating something because you would feel guilty throwing it away?

FAT TO FREE ACTION PLAN

List out all the scenarios when you eat that may be due to other reasons besides hunger.

You should no longer choose to put food in your mouth unless you can determine that you're truly hungry. Don't let yourself get "hangry." You want to avoid situations where your emotions are high and you feel overwhelmed. But if you've done the activity above and determined the signs that indicate when your body is hungry, you'll learn to eat only when you need to.

A note for Type 2 diabetics: During this time, test your blood sugar often and include that in your observations. You may be surprised by what you think your body is telling you and what is really going on.

Here are some tips to keep you from eating when your body isn't truly hungry.

◇ Always keep water with you. What feels like hunger is often thirst.

◇ Chew sugarless gum.

◇ Take a walk.

◇ Call a friend.

◇ Review your goals and why you are making changes.

◇ Get busy—do a household chore that you have been putting off.

◇ Spend time with a loved one.

◇ Listen to a podcast or read a book that is in line with your goals.

Food is everywhere, so how do you end this toxic relationship? One step at a time, just like you learned.

FREE: MARCH 23, 2018

I want to eat. Eating right now would feel good. I don't care if it's temporary. Okay, I do care. I'm just being a drama queen. Guess I haven't kicked that habit yet. I crack myself up.

Life is difficult. All the feelings stirring around in me. I cry a lot. Nobody seems to understand. I guess that's okay as this is my crap. It feels like it's oozing out of my pores. Gross!

Thank goodness there's not an apple pie in the house right now because I'd be tempted to eat it. Ugh, I know, I know...the food would only make me feel worse. I'm going to take a shower and get a good night's sleep, then start again tomorrow.

YOUR LESSON:
Recognize when you're hungry.
Recognize when you're full.

FAT TO FREE ACTION PLAN

Choose a day when you'll observe being hungry. Sit alone and observe what your body is doing. Remember, you're in control. Practice many times. Don't worry, you won't starve.

Push your hunger a little bit beyond the normal stage so you can hear the noises in your stomach, experience your mood and your body's responses. Write it all down. What is your body's response to hunger? Did you experience any emotions? How can you identify the difference between a hunger cue and an emotional cue?

You are thinking about so many behaviors and making new choices. Let's make sure you are not expecting perfection.

CHAPTER EIGHT: STARTING OVER AGAIN

FAT: AUGUST 2, 2013

Doctor tells me I am a walking time bomb. I feel it. I'm scared. I'm disgusted. Time to take care of ME. How? Less stress. Less control. Breathe. How?

FEELING WORTHY

All those years ago, I knew I needed to take action, but I didn't know how. I spent years in counseling to analyze my life. I dissected my past to determine the source of my low self-worth. The bottom line was that I wasn't willing to make any real changes to care for myself and have the life I wanted. And self-sabotage was always easier than admitting the hard stuff or doing the difficult work.

From the past few chapters, you already know the drill—your choices are yours and you must take action. But let's talk about how self-sabotage can get in the way and the tools you need to battle it.

Think back about times in your life when you felt unworthy. It could be many small items piled up over the years or something big that happened once. Mine was a combination of both.

In my early twenties, I worked at a retirement community. I was the Dining Room Supervisor, which involved hiring and managing more than 20 waitstaff members. It was a great job where I discovered my love for helping others while using business skills I inherited from my grandfather, Doodad.

Each year, they would have a contest to identify the "Best of the Best": the employee who demonstrated the organization's values and always went above and beyond. First, each facility voted for their best, then those candidates would compete at the national level.

I was nominated because my efforts had resulted in many positive changes and because I had developed a training program and built a team of people who received excellent feedback from the residents. I was honored to be nominated and excited to be part of the award process. But I was also embarrassed. The negative voices screamed in my head, *Why would a fat girl win such an honor?* The anticipation of a spotlight on me was difficult. I worked hard for it. I was uncomfortable.

After the votes were tallied, I was called into a small private dining room with the other nominees. They called my name. The community had voted for me! I felt excited and proud...for a minute. But then I saw a look of disgust from someone I admired. She said the only reason I had won was because I had such a large staff who had voted for me. Ouch.

A cloud passed over me and immediately stole all my excitement. I added this incident to the ever-growing pile of reasons I felt unworthy. Even though I was full of fear over the attention the award was going to bring, the recognition felt good. But I let her steal my joy. I should have held my head high, as I did feel worthy until I let someone take it away.

The process continued, and a few months later I received the award for not just for the local facility but for the nationwide company. Interestingly, the woman who made the comment had led the campaign to help me win at the national level. I remember how anxious I was speaking at each event. The parties were uncomfortable and I could not block out the voice in my head saying this must be a mistake. I let the negativity in and walked away believing I was not worthy.

This all happened during a time that I was at my heaviest weight. My chins (yes, I had many) were at their largest, and I was so uncomfortable that I would rarely sit without pulling whatever shirt or dress I was wearing up over my nose so that nobody could see them. I could feel them hitting the top of my chest over my collarbones. It was a constant reminder that I was uncomfortable in my skin.

This award ceremony and the pictures from it led me to take drastic measures in my early twenties. I had liposuction surgery on my face. I have no idea how I convinced a doctor to do the surgery with my being at least 130 pounds overweight, but I did.

I actually don't regret that drastic measure. In fact, it wasn't long after the surgery that I took off for six weeks to a fat camp to experience another failed attempt to feel better about my body. I have done it all.

IDENTIFYING SELF-SABOTAGE

That woman's response wasn't about me; it was all about her. So often we let others define our worth. But nobody gets to decide your worth or your happiness, or steal your joy from you. I was worthy of the award. If my staff hadn't felt that way, they wouldn't have taken the time to vote.

Self-sabotage is a buzzword that gets thrown around in this journey without much consideration to owning the behavior. The simplest way to identify self-sabotage is to ask yourself some questions.

◇ Does one side of me want one thing and another side want something else?

◇ Are my behaviors (choices) creating problems that interfere with my long-term goals?

Your self-sabotaging may not only affect your weight-loss goals; it could also be showing up in your relationships or professional career. Once you start down the rabbit hole of self-sabotage, it's hard to get out—but not impossible.

The two most common signs of self-sabotage are procrastination and self-medication with alcohol or comfort eating. Sound familiar? If those don't resonate, there are other more subtle signs, including:

◇ Fear of success

◇ Overthinking when you face too many options

◇ Giving up when tasks get difficult

◇ Letting others take your time when you should be doing something else

◇ Avoiding work on a project by doing other trivial tasks

◇ Talking negatively to yourself

◇ Not making sleep a priority.

How many of these do you identify with?

FAT TO FREE ACTION PLAN

Take a minute to reflect and write about where any lack of worthiness has come from. Examine how that feeling plays a role in your own self-sabotage.

Did you ever want something badly but were so filled with fear that you found excuses to guarantee that you'd never get it? This kind of procrastination once again puts you in the role of victim when life doesn't work out your way. This can be true even when you don't feel like you've made a conscious decision to sabotage.

We say we are too busy, we choose to be lazy, or we convince ourselves that we are not capable. But the truth is that procrastination is just being unwilling to do something, and your reasons are ultimately all excuses.

Procrastination is only one form of self-sabotage. You may find yourself stuck because you're comfortable with what is familiar, or because your fear of rejection is stronger than your desire for success. If you're fighting against familiarity, it can be as easy as slowing down, assessing the situation, and taking a deep breath. Trying new experiences can be uncomfortable, but that's where the joy happens.

Are you willing to stop sabotaging and start choosing success? Change your language.

"I am worthy. I am willing!"

Don't let others define your worth. Stop self-sabotaging and start choosing success. There it is again—choice.

You're fighting against old, deep thoughts and memories. The greatest defense against this is planning. Having a plan and committing to moving through it allows less time for thoughts of fear or unworthiness.

FREE: JANUARY 1, 2018

Well, that was a hard year. I'm most proud of finally making myself a priority and choosing to start getting healthy. Others aren't so proud of me. I want to bring a better me to all parts of my life. I'm exhausted from half-ass living for so long.

I am finally taking off my fat armor. It has gotten too heavy. Uncomfortable is okay and, in fact, interesting at times. I'm not so sure about all of this, but I keep moving forward. I feel done with the past. I feel done with the fat. New year. Excited to see what choosing me will lead to.

> *YOUR LESSON:*
> *Stop making excuses and*
> *sabotaging your own life.*

FAT TO FREE ACTION PLAN

What inspires you? Surround yourself with ideas and messages to remind you what choices you want to make to keep you on track with reaching your goals. Every day, you will be faced with messages coming at you from many sources. You can decide what those messages are. Are there words that speak to you? What at-a-glance reminder will keep your mind full of positive thoughts?

Here are some ideas to get you started.

◇ Jewelry: I have a bracelet that says *Unstoppable* and another that says *Overcomer*. Find a charm that speaks to you, or wear your children's birthstones if they are part of your why.

◇ Magnets: Having a reminder on the refrigerator is a great last line of defense.

◇ Pictures: Change the screensavers or backgrounds on your computer and phone. Hang photos around your house to remember your why.

◇ Stickers: One that relates to my goals reads "Go outside." It reminds me that I want to be active and also of how good it feels to take a few minutes for myself. Put stickers on your water bottle, your journal, your laptop—wherever you'll see them often.

You can also set yourself up with reminders through podcasts, social media, and accountability groups. Listen to a podcast on a morning walk to set the tone for the day. Follow social media sites that are in line with your goals.

Mute the people, brands, and pages that don't serve your new lifestyle.

Have fun with these! Find a new coffee mug that starts your day with a smile. An apron with a little humor or a little confidence boost will remind you to make good choices in the kitchen. A keychain will catch your eye throughout the day. You control these messages—stay positive.

Fill your life with positive items and positive people.

CHAPTER NINE:
DON'T DO THIS ALONE

FAT: JANUARY 16, 2006

I wasn't honest with him. I didn't tell him what was on my mind. I'm pretty sure that even if I had, I'd still be disappointed and hurt. What would I say if I were honest? I'm lonely. Tomorrow I'll stop hiding behind my fat. I will live. I will feel. I will let go. I will live in the moment. Tomorrow I will take care of my body by giving it proper water, food, and exercise.

HIDING IN PLAIN SIGHT

I wonder how many "tomorrows" there are in all of my journals? I chose to share this entry because it highlights the extent of my hiding, the results from it, and my continued desire to change. I didn't want others to know how I was feeling. They saw my pain with my body getting bigger and bigger, but I rarely opened up about what was behind it all.

My immediate family members are close, and I know I can count on any one of them to come running if I call. I also have several people in my life who I consider extended family. I have good friends. I've been in romantic relationships. But I've always chosen to keep most of them at arm's length.

In fact, I bet many of them will learn more about me by reading this book than they knew before. They may have suspected, but most of them never asked and I never talked about it. As a result, I felt isolated and alone, lacked intimate connections, and had many failed relationships. My trust issues are extensive. I know now that this was all a result of my choices.

I also know I am incredibly lucky. Even though I've struggled to bring my true self to the table, I still have a handful of loved ones (you know who you are) who are reliable and will no doubt make contact after reading this. Their love has been unconditional from the beginning.

I hope you know the kind—when life hits you in the gut, they show up for support. When life deserves a celebration, they join in. Or when it's just been too long since they heard from you, they check in to make sure you're okay.

When Sophie's dad died, I learned a lot about the people in my life. More importantly, I learned about love, forgiveness, and the importance of communication. I learned that I'm terrible at asking for help and even worse at accepting it.

Someone suggested to me that Tim's death was a gift, and I was outraged at first. I wasn't ready to hear it. The journey of grief was so painful, and watching my daughter navigate that, I was unable to hear what they were trying to tell me. Through this experience, some relationships in my life were healed and others didn't survive. The greatest gift, however, was that I realized how precious life is and how tomorrow is never promised.

I've been blessed with many tomorrows, and it was time to stop wasting them. I had to take advantage of every single one. This was an extreme example of a life challenge where I had 100% control over how to respond. I was also still early in my journey, so even though my response needed some work, the lessons I learned were pivotal. I worked so hard not to go down a rabbit hole of regret.

If you're making similar choices with your loved ones, I suggest you add this to the top of your action list: Start bringing your true self to all your relationships—the good, the bad, and the ugly. The people in your life who are there out of love will remain, and you'll experience deeper and more rewarding relationships. You will find the results you want just by being true to yourself. You don't need to manipulate anything. You no longer need to hide your true self.

Be real. Be you. Be vulnerable.

Not sure where to start? I can help with that.

PUT YOURSELF OUT THERE

You may have a desire to hide how you're working on weight loss (yet again). You think about how many times you've announced a new plan only to be back to your old choices within a week. You're likely hesitant because countless times before you've declared, "This is the time!"

Let that go. This journey is about choosing differently so you get different results. I say throw caution to the wind and tell everyone! You'll need all the support you can get, so stand tall and own what you're doing.

You'll run into naysayers, people who try to convince you to make different choices. But when anyone tries to knock you off track, remember that their negativity is more about them than you. You might be surprised when your family says things like, "Now you're too thin," or they encourage you to eat junk food because "you've earned it." But by now, you know that food is not to be used as a reward.

How do you handle these unwanted comments from others? Smile and walk away. Don't invest time or energy into trying to convince them of what you know to be true. You may be pleasantly surprised when they come back around and ask for advice. The hard part is letting go of the desire to change them or make them choose what you're doing. But it's not your business or your concern. Lead in love, serve as a positive role model, and they will follow.

You're embarking on a journey that will result in many changes to your body and in your life as well. Have you considered what this might mean for others in your life? My advice for these conversations is not to ask for permission, or even approval. You don't need it. This is your life. This time will be different, including the conversations you'll have with your loved ones.

THE TALK

When most of us learn about a change happening to someone else, we often think, *How will this impact my life?* If you're married or in a relationship, you need to anticipate that this is what your partner is thinking, even if they're unable to express that to you. Once you've determined your goals and mapped out daily objectives, share it all with your loved ones. This is significant not only so they can support you, but also to give them tools they'll need to do that effectively.

When talking to your loved ones, it can be helpful to explain your objectives and what a typical day will look like for you. It's possible they will react with a great deal of negativity. Listen to them. Realize that you've just cast a spotlight on their life and poor choices as well, so they may feel judged. Accept them for where they are in their own journey.

Then realize their choices are not yours to make. You're only responsible for what you do. You've decided to take control and be healthy. If they want to do the same, that's great, but it's completely up to them to decide. You might inspire them, but they will have to do the work just like you are.

Be specific when you ask friends and family for help. Don't just say, "If you see me eating badly, remind me to stop." You need to give clear actions they can take to assist you in that moment. Maybe you need them to take you by the hand and say, "Let's go for a walk." Maybe you want them to suggest you leave the kitchen for a bit until cravings subside. You have to define exactly what help looks like for you.

If you need to rid your house of all junk food or avoid eating out for a while, tell them that's what you'll need to succeed. Don't assume anyone will know exactly what you need as you're establishing all these new habits. If your needs change or you find something that works or doesn't, be honest. They want to help you; they likely just don't know how.

Share details. Your loved ones don't understand your emotional eating and might resist making adjustments in their world just so you won't be tempted to grab some cookies. They need to know just how desperate the situation is for you. This requires a level of vulnerability you've probably worked to avoid for most of your life. To make it even harder, you have to do it at a time when food is still your source of comfort. Learn from my mistakes and be vulnerable anyway.

Communication is imperative. If you want different results from your loved ones, you have to approach it differently. Reassure them. Be honest that you don't know what this is going to look like, but you're asking them to stand by you. They may not want to at first. They may wonder why this time will be any different. Don't let this discourage you.

Start making changes, and eventually most will jump on board. Give them time to process and to realize this change in your life will actually lead to good for them as well. Remember, it's your responsibility to fix your life; you just want them to come along for the ride. You'll do it regardless of their response...one pound at a time.

You may be surprised at what people will say to you on this journey. For me, it was interesting that for years people had never told me to stop shoving donuts in my face, but when I started eating real food and drinking a gallon of water every day, everyone suddenly had an opinion, and it wasn't what you might think. It was not all helpful and supportive; they had a lot of judgment about what I was doing to get the weight off.

Set your intentions, your goals, and your daily objectives and trust the process. Any judgment sent your way is not your problem. It is about them. Become comfortable with smiling, nodding, and saying nothing.

FREE: FEBRUARY 18, 2020

Tonight I sat with new friends and laughed harder than I had in a long time. The greatest part was that we laughed at ourselves. Past pains have healed, and I'm now able to share them with others who understand. There was no judgment. There was understanding. Coming on this trip was out of my comfort zone, but as I keep learning, being uncomfortable leads to the greatest joy. My tribe is growing.

YOUR LESSON:
Be vulnerable, present your true self, and build your support system.

FAT TO FREE ACTION PLAN

Who is your support system?

1. List at least three people you would like support from on this journey.

2. Determine what that support looks like specifically—at home, at work, in your hobbies, and on the weekends.

3. Contact each person, share your story, and ask for the specific help you need to be successful.

You are doing great and building strength around you. Now it is time to take down some more barriers.

CHAPTER TEN:
OH, SO MANY LIES

FAT: FEBRUARY 22, 2006

The truth about the truth—it hurts! So lie. The perfect motto about my feelings.

September 4, 2013

So, so excited until I got on the scale! Pissed. Back up to 240. WTF? Discouraged. (Note: My food log right after this reflects that I went out to eat at 8:45 p.m. and had a steak, sweet potato fries, and veggies.)

WAS IT YOU? OR WAS IT ME?

Certainly, there are judgment and discrimination toward overweight people. We may start a weight-loss journey many times only to gain the pounds back, so most people don't believe we're even trying. The common belief or explanation is that we're just lazy. When a situation requires sitting close, like in a movie theater or on an airplane, we cause an inconvenience.

We create a disturbance in any kind of small space—a grocery store aisle or an elevator.

When I declared that I was going to try one more diet, I had a gastric bypass surgeon laugh at me. When I did start to get healthy, a pharmacist asked why I was cutting back on my diabetes medications. When I told him, his response was, "You'll be back." Interactions like these can certainly justify my desire to look down, to avoid eye contact or conversation, to avoid having to explain myself.

The first journal entry in this chapter is far more honest than the second one. My life was full of lies for everyone, but the most damaging were the ones I told myself. That I needed fat to protect me against uncomfortable eye contact or vulnerability in relationships at any level—including sex—and most poignantly, sharing my true self and putting my heart at risk of being broken. The lie I told myself was that fat could push people away and protect me from getting hurt. Wrong.

Beyond this most damaging lie, I repeated numerous others. You can see it in the second journal entry, in the way I seem so surprised and angry when my weight was back up again. At that time, I didn't know how to fuel my body correctly. Regardless, most weight-loss attempts were half-assed and followed by exclamations that "I just don't understand why this isn't working!" I wasn't actually doing the work. I was lying to myself and everyone around me.

Eventually I hit rock bottom and decided to change my life. I stopped lying to myself and playing a victim. I took real action with no excuses. Once I started to shed pounds, I began to look up and look around. I was greeted with smiles and well wishes. People were more willing to greet me, interact with me, and help me out.

At first it was uncomfortable, but soon I began to find joy in it. My day would be lifted by a simple hello or an offer to reach something for me off a high shelf. The genuine interaction I had quietly craved for years was becoming less scary and more enjoyable. I found myself wanting to give that same recognition and affirmation to others. Even more satisfying than being seen is finding someone who may be looking down, hiding, or needing help but is too scared to ask. I know how that feels.

So was it me or was it you?

My answer to the question now: both. I have no doubt that for most of my life I chose to avoid eye contact, social inter-action, and anything that could be defined as intimacy. But it was also easy to blame others for avoiding me first and to blame society for labeling me an inconvenience or a disturbance. But placing all that blame is a convenient lie I told myself to continue my victim role.

Now I accept and take ownership of my choices, past and present. If other people want to look away, that's about them and their choices, not me. For so many years, I actively looked down and away. But thankfully, one day I was ready to accept my space in the world, make a change I could control, and look up.

THE LIES YOU TELL YOURSELF

The lies you're living and telling, not only to yourself but also to others in your life, will do lasting damage and can lead to endless hurt. It's time to stop. I rarely rely on tough love, but this warrants it. Sometimes we all just need a swifter nudge. Stop it. Now.

Your fat is not helping you. Your fat is not protecting you. I believe in my heart that you know that. You continue to hide behind the fat as the more comfortable route right now. But take a leap of faith, and you'll quickly realize that the road untraveled is far easier than the one you're on right now.

You may still be struggling with my use of the word *fat*. It could be considered harsh. But it's the truth, the bold truth, and if you're here to make real changes, you have to accept it and own it. It's time to start living in the truth. I chose to precisely *because* it's uncomfortable. I needed to be uncomfortable and so do you.

Doctors, family, friends, and coworkers might tiptoe around the reality of your being overweight. You can't waste time tiptoeing anymore. It's time to own the reality, because if you don't, you're starting this process off with yet another lie. Nothing else has knocked you into making new choices, so maybe putting the truth out there will.

There is an excess of fat on your body, and it's there because of your choices.

What is your fat doing for you? How are all your lies impacting your life? Maybe you're missing out on being a part of your family members' lives or unable to spend quality time with your children. Are your relationships based on false pretenses because you're not bringing the real YOU to the table? How is it impacting your sex life? You're probably missing out on meeting great people and having new experiences.

You're sick and shortening your life span. Your body hurts and you're slowly killing yourself. You hurt physically and emotionally and are spreading hurt to the ones you love.

Worst of all, if you have children, you're teaching them this behavior. And one day—if they haven't already—they will start to use food as their comfort, entertainment, reward, or cure for boredom.

The lies must stop and the work has to start. Identify the lies in your life and start speaking the truth. It's time to look up and start living life as your true self.

FREE: SEPTEMBER 9, 2019

Convincing myself that my hurt and my emptiness were due to everyone else and taking no personal accountability has landed me alone again. I sit here tonight sad and full of regret. I'm choosing to feel it. I'm not eating it. I continue to find blessings in this journey. I don't know where the road will lead, but I have hope and believe that it will be only more beautiful because of my new choices.

My friends said that it's time for me to date. Oh, I don't know about that yet, but the difference between now and 10 years ago when I was dating... I get to bring the better me to the table. I'm good with that!

YOUR LESSON:
Stop lying to yourself.

FAT TO FREE ACTION PLAN

What are the lies you've been telling yourself?

1. List at least three. I'm guessing that if you put some time into it, you'll come up with even more. It doesn't have to relate to your being overweight or your relationship with food. This is an opportunity to take a step back and do a thorough analysis of lies you want to own and let go.

2. Once you've written out all the lies, you need to write the truth. The truth is the reality that you are scared to acknowledge because it oftentimes means ownership of choices you have made, and that hurts. By writing out the truth, you start to get rid of the layers of emotional fat that you have been hiding behind. It is the excuses you tell yourself and others. Some examples of lies you might tell yourself followed by the truth could be...

   ◆ My fat is protecting me. > My fat is killing me.

   ◆ Being fat runs in my family. > I'm fat because of what I eat.

   ◆ I'm the happy fat person. > I'm faking being happy.

Now that you are dealing with some truth, it is time to learn how to break some of those habits you've been holding on to for so many years.

CHAPTER ELEVEN: BREAKING HABITS

FAT: JUNE 10, 2007

Life is what you make it. I am scared. I keep avoiding my reality. I feel so alone. I don't want to get hurt anymore. I don't want to get rejected anymore, so I avoid it. I choose to be alone.

BE PRESENT

We all have habits. We tend to do what we have done before. Think about your typical day. Do you remember brushing your teeth? Do you remember the drive to work or the store? Your day is filled with tasks like putting on shoes, locking the front door, closing the garage—all done without thought. These are habits.

Does it apply to your eating as well? Do you remember any thought process before grabbing a piece of candy and eating it? Do you find yourself in a drive-thru, looking in the pantry, eating the cookies on the table, or opening another can of Diet Coke without any thought?

My journals are filled with emotions and feelings I wanted to stop. When I learned how much of any given day was filled with mindless habits, I realized that if I changed some of those habits, I'd start seeing change in the corresponding feelings. This became an indirect approach to making change, but I needed something I could hold on to. I needed to stop wallowing in all those emotions and have something tangible I could do.

Action steps would equal results—an incredibly appealing prospect. Changing some of my habits like eating when I was bored were small steps, but it sure felt good to finally have something I could focus on. I was finally taking charge and taking action.

Are you ready to feel some success toward digging out of this rabbit hole?

There are two ways you can manage your habits as they relate to eating. For one, you can identify a negative habit and actively work to change it. The second way is to add in some good new habits like drinking water, getting good sleep, and fueling your body with real food. With both of these angles working together, you can find success.

RECOGNIZE HABITS

Ready to change some habits? Let's use the example of snacking in the evening as a habit you want to change. First, change is hard and makes us uncomfortable. Cut yourself some slack. This is not going to be as simple as reading a few paragraphs to change all your habits and get skinny. But this is a beautiful journey, so take a deep breath, buckle up, and get ready for the ride. You have some work to do, and it will take effort each day.

Every habit has a function. If you can identify the function, you'll be able to start changing your response.

The first identifier is the **signal.** In our example of snacking in the evening, think about why you end up there in the first place. Boredom is a common answer. So the signal is that you're bored, and you start looking for ways to resolve that feeling.

The second identifier is the **action,** or your response to the signal. You're bored so you get off the couch and walk into the kitchen to snack. You're not actually hungry.

The third identifier of a habit is the **reward** your action delivers. If you're bored and choose to eat, the reward might be that you just passed time to avoid doing items like household chores. I mean, we all like to avoid the laundry and dishes. For me, this usually meant I could go to bed.

Now that you know the makeup of habits, it's time to deal with the problem—changing them. For each habit, look at the signal and action to adjust your behaviors. In the example above, what could you do instead of eating when you're bored? Well, the list is endless.

FAT TO FREE ACTION PLAN

Make a list of non-food activities you can do when you're bored. It may sound elementary, but your action is a habit without thought. To change the habit, you need to be prepared with a tool to help you in the moment. You should do this exercise for each habit you're working to change.

Make it easy on yourself and have that list ready. The signals won't go away—you'll still be bored from time to time. What you can choose to change is your action and your reward.

From the activity in Chapter Nine, you should have at least one person you can rely on to support you. Who is on this journey with you? When you're working on breaking habits and old ways start to creep back in, or the negative voice is loud and pushing you toward the kitchen, you need to lean on your support.

But remember, you need to be specific and tell others what will be helpful to you at the moment you're struggling. If they see you in the kitchen mindlessly staring into the pantry, what is one statement they could say to help redirect your action? Mine was, "Maybe you should review your list of options that are more in line with your health goals."

Again, this is not a quick fix. But change is change no matter how small. The fact that you're here reading this and learning how to end your toxic relationship with food—that is a huge step toward positive change. Don't expect it all to happen overnight. You'll only get discouraged, and that can result in you turning back to old habits. If you take deliberate steps toward your goals each day, you will be successful. One day, you'll start seeing your new positive actions becoming habits.

Perfection is a ridiculous expectation for anyone. Allow for stumbles. Yes, stumbles—not mistakes. It takes practice. When it happens, be graceful to yourself. There is no time for the shame and guilt we so often pile on our shoulders. Here is yet another opportunity where you have 100% control of how you respond. You deserve the same grace you would give to anyone else you witness struggling. Then recommit and try again.

It is no different than when a child is trying to ride a bike. When they fall, they have to pop up and continue to try. We all cheer them on and even applaud every effort. We teach them how they can do better and say, "Do it again." We do not let them give up. They learn from each stumble, and eventually, the training wheels come off, and there's no stopping them.

As you begin to change your habits, your mindset will also change and you'll start noticing those around you living in habit mode, not even realizing they have the power to change it. You might even start analyzing and judging them.

Be kind. Be understanding. Stay in your own lane. Remember, not so long ago, you were in the same boat. Others have their own journeys, and they just may not be ready yet. Use this opportunity to continue to self-reflect and identify more habits you want to address.

FREE: JANUARY 23, 2018

The past six months have been one heck of a ride. The lessons have been overwhelming. The pain and loss hurts. I have to stand strong for Sophie. But this is not comfortable. Tim died. My relationship is over. My dad is here in the ICU. Feeling all of this is hard, but each day I walk out from this hospital and I feel strong. The blessings and the lessons are plentiful.

I even packed my meals and water to have with me at the hospital. Cafeteria food has been calling my name, but I'm ignoring it. I'm proud of myself. Weird. One day, one step at a time. My future is full of new and different and I'm scared. I'm ready for it. I will be okay. Weird.

> **YOUR LESSON:**
> *Break your bad habits. Build new ones. Actively protect yourself, your goals, and your health.*

FAT TO FREE ACTION PLAN

1. List the bad habits you are ready to break.

2. Choose the top three you want to work on first.

3. Take each one of those and identify the signal, action, and reward. What will your new habits look like after you make the changes you desire?

4. Now pick the top one that you're going to commit to work on for the next 30 days. Develop your goal, objectives, and safeguards to ensure they happen, along with rewards for your success. Make sure part of your plan is to have your list of activities you can do instead of your habit.

Is fear stopping you from changing your habits? Let's take a look at that and help you push through it.

BONUS TOOL BELT STRENGTH

"I can't tell you how many times I've heard someone say they wish they had more willpower to be able to quit sugar. But here's the thing: It's an actual physical addiction, and the food industry strives to get us hooked on sugar. It's not about willpower; it's about biochemistry."

— Mark Hyman, MD

Food is everywhere, and that makes this change infinitely more difficult. It doesn't help that the food industry makes everything enticing and addictive by adding sugar.

What does your life need to look like to prevent yourself from falling back into old habits? Identify exactly what you need to protect the new you. Don't rely on willpower; it will eventually get the best of you.

Here are some safeguards you can use to avoid stumbling and falling back into old habits.

◇ Keep no junk food in the house.

◇ Schedule work meetings so they are not associated with food. (This is much less of a concern now with the current pandemic. The situation actually provides an excellent opportunity to change your behavior before you do get back to having face-to-face meetings and gatherings.)

◇ When someone wants to meet with you, suggest a meeting spot that helps you avoid temptation. This can be uncomfortable at first, but you'll feel empowered when you start standing up for yourself.

If you're unable to avoid the situation, take charge by planning ahead. Most restaurants have a menu online, so you can decide which healthy options you'll order before you arrive. This prevents you from even having to open the menu while you're there so you can avoid being tempted by unhealthy food.

The same can work for coffee meetings as well. Many coffee shops are starting to offer sugar-free options. Or you could order coffee but bring your own mug with whatever you like to mix in from home instead of the syrups and sugars typically available. Or just drink water.

◇ Don't go to social functions or food shopping when you're hungry.

◇ Bring water and chew gum when grocery shopping.

Even better, order online and pick up your groceries at the curb. This is the most wonderful service! When you shop online, it's much easier to stay focused and only pick the items on your list. You avoid temptation from all the goodies and ads within the store. And you know what else? Your grocery bill is lower—win and win! If you can afford to pay a little more, you can even have groceries delivered to your home.

◇ Meal prep on weekends.

This is key to success. If you don't have to think about making a meal and can just grab what you know to be healthy, you'll avoid getting too hungry and reacting with your emotions. The less time you have to think about it in the moment that you need fuel, the better your decisions will be. Set aside two hours on the weekends to prepare several meals and make your week much easier.

◇ Plan, plan, plan!

You should plan out meals in terms of your weekly activities. What meetings or events do you have next week? Who are you spending time with?

We are all productive and tend to be running from one thing to the next. Running kids around to after-school activities and taking care of our homes all while trying to spend time with friends and family.

When you plan your week, include how to take care of yourself. Going to be stuck in the car driving? Bring a meal with you. Maybe you have a family gathering that is late in the day. Make sure you don't go hungry so you are less tempted by sugary foods.

FAT TO FREE ACTION PLAN

1. What safeguards do you need to have in place? Once you've identified those, document them and post it somewhere easy to find. Writing them out is important because you can easily slip back into old habits and scenarios that don't support your objectives.

2. Share your safeguards with members of your household, friends, and even coworkers. For example, if you and a coworker have always gone out to drinks after work and you know you

need to stop, that should be on the list. The two of you can go to a movie, take a hike, or go shopping. Talk to anyone who is impacted and bring them on the journey.

3. Brainstorm together some other activities you can enjoy. Is there a class you can take after work instead?

Remember that the people in your life just want to know how your changes will impact them. If you replace the old behavior with something new, you likely won't get too much pushback. Taking this step and sharing it with others isn't selfish; it's critical.

CHAPTER TWELVE: EMBRACING THE FEAR

FAT: FEBRUARY 9, 2006

I don't like myself. I give up as soon as I get scared. As soon as I heard "Wow, you look good," I stopped—fear set in. I'm treating my body poorly, making bad choices. Why? I want to beat this. How?

WHAT DO YOU FEAR?

Words associated with fear include apprehension, dread, terror, angst, anxiety, horror, panic, and tension. Sounds about right. Merriam-Websters' definition of fear is "an unpleasant often strong emotion caused by anticipation or awareness of danger."

The list of experiences I missed out on due to fear is long. There was a period in my life when I found it easy and convenient to blame everything on work. I often said that I would show up and then skipped out. I missed camping adventures, joining friends for gatherings, and even vacations with my family. I was exhausted and hiding.

One time, my parents took Sophie to the Oregon coast, and I had said I could not go due to work, which at the time I convinced myself was true, but the reality was that by staying home I could sit on the couch, watch television, and sleep. And during that trip, Sophie lost her first tooth. I missed it.

I missed so much. It takes a lot of energy not to spiral into regret.

What fears do you have? What does that have to do with weight loss? Believe it or not, this is an imperative aspect of your journey. If you're not ready to face your fears, you won't get beyond them.

Are you ready? If you aren't, it's okay. You can absolutely be fearful of facing them. Everything will happen in its own time. But I encourage you to keep reading, because learning how to address them may be enough to get you moving forward.

Did you know that fear is an opportunity to develop courage? What you accomplish in life is often a result of how you respond to it. Think about one that you've addressed head-on in the past and how you felt afterward.

We often believe others are successful because they seem to have no fear. That's just not accurate. You don't get to throw yourself into a victim role over experiencing it. Fear never goes away. You have to accept it as a reality. Everyone experiences it. It doesn't matter how strong someone seems. Nobody is navigating through life without apprehension or concern. They simply have tools to face it and push through it.

When I shared some of my fears, I was often told they were just excuses; they were not met with understanding. As you learned earlier, you need to drop the excuses. It's assumed when we are fat that we should want to be healthy so badly that fears are not warranted. At a minimum, we should be able to push right past them, stop making excuses, and get healthy. This is true to an extent, but on some level, these were also genuine fears coming from someone who had been fat for a long time.

Fear and excuses often go hand in hand. I'm here to tell you that those fears and others you have are real and valid. By identifying them now and taking some of the emotional charge out of them, you'll be able to navigate through them as they arise throughout your journey.

You should do one scary activity every day. Start small. I'm not talking about playing with spiders or jumping out of a plane. How about trying some of those activities you stopped doing because you were overweight and hiding from the world? Have you feared making eye contact, shopping at a certain store, playing with your children, or riding a bike? I have no doubt your list is as long as mine. Here are some other questions that may be swirling around in the fear part of your brain.

◊ Will there be new expectations of me? Now that I'm skinny, will people want me to do physical activities that I'm truly not interested in?

◊ Will people find me attractive? And not the fake kind of attraction where they tell me what I want to hear just for sex. Will there be real intimacy where they get to know the real me?

◊ Who will I be? I fear losing my identity. Are there parts of my life that will change because I am no longer fat?

◊ What if I fail again?

⋄ What if I'm not good enough even after I lose weight?

Identifying your fears about losing weight (and anything else) and learning how to navigate through them is a vital step so you're aware of them and not subconsciously avoiding opportunities out of habit. Sorry, the bad news is that the fear doesn't go away; the good news is that you can manage it. You are taking what seems big and scary and attacking it little by little. By doing this work up front, you'll start to notice you're okay and begin to feel more confident.

FAT TO FREE ACTION PLAN

1. Write down your fears and limiting beliefs.

2. Then rewrite them with confidence instead of fear.

For example...

FEAR: "I'm afraid that I'm going to get more attention once I have lost the weight."

REWRITE: "I decide what I do and who I hang out with. While I may discover that others want to give me more attention, I get to decide when I will receive it."

FACE IT

My fear of horses started when I was in elementary school and our family was on vacation. I begged my parents to let us ride. When we were in the arena, something spooked my horse. It took off running, and I believed it was going to jump the fence onto a busy street. I was screaming. Thankfully, the horse stopped at the fence and I was able to climb off of her safely.

I let that experience keep me off horses for more than 40 years. It was on my list of adventures to try again, and I finally got the opportunity in 2020. A friend invited me out to her house to begin the process of facing my fear.

Driving out to her house, I had some of my typical signs of fear, including sweaty palms and a sick stomach. But I told myself that I was going through with it. I think I felt comfort just knowing I could back out if I wanted to.

The horses seemed huge and strong, but they were also gentle. My friend was kind and knew of my fear, so she walked me through the process slowly. She assured me that day was just about getting comfortable around the horse and she wouldn't let go of the reigns.

We rode for two hours, and it truly was not until the end that I began to relax a little bit. I almost said that I wanted to try to ride without her holding on, but I didn't. I knew that I would stick to my habit of trying everything three times, so that is my goal for the next time.

The fear did not go away. I chose to feel it and stay on that horse. The jury is still out on my feelings about horses, but I do know I will go again.

When you're experiencing fear, you cannot just think your way through it. Yes, you need to be mindful and aware, but sometimes you should just feel whatever it is and move on. Your analysis of the what-ifs or the whys doesn't in any way diminish what is happening and often makes it worse. Don't work against it—feel it. Face it.

Have you seen any horror movie where the actors are always running from what scares them? Of course, they run because it keeps the suspense going. What would happen if instead they turned and faced whatever it is? The fear would be gone much faster. Not entertaining for a movie, but this is your real life we're talking about.

Stop running from it. Turn around and deal with it. Get on to happier storylines.

RULE OF THREE

Then you must practice it. I know, another difficult suggestion. You're probably thinking, "I'm scared of something and you want me to do it again and again?" Well, yes. More precisely, I want you to do it at least three times. This is something I learned from my dear friend Jamie when Sophie was young, and I've done it ever since.

One of the first times I put this into practice was riding a roller coaster. It was especially nerve-racking because I was still fat at the time and wondering whether the safety bar was going to lock in place over my large stomach. I remember standing in line and feeling my insides shake and palms sweat. But I was determined. In order to keep moving forward in line, I would look at all the little kids who were excited to go on the ride and tell myself, "If they can do it, so can I."

Thankfully, the bar locked into place. (Although in that moment I was secretly wishing it wouldn't, as it would give me the excuse to get out.) The roller coaster was tame in comparison to some that are out there, with a typical tall incline and many ups and downs after. No going upside down.

I scream-laughed uncontrollably as we climbed the first hill. Once we came over the edge and headed down, it was all screaming. My heart was racing, and my palms and entire body were drenched with sweat. Despite all of this discomfort, I did notice a bit of thrill and even fun. That is what helped me climb on for a second ride.

And though that next time there was some screaming, there was much more laughter. I noted that I was okay and even enjoyed the ride a little bit. The third time I had fun. No shaking, and my screams had turned to laughter. My current to-do list includes riding a roller coaster again now that I am healthy.

When you have to do something that scares you, try it three times before deciding how you feel. The first time, you likely won't experience much beyond anxiety from your built-up and likely overinflated fear. This will prove you can survive the discomfort. The second time, you can start to look around and experience adventure and newness. The third time, you'll have your eyes wide open because you know what's coming. At that point, you can decide whether it's something you enjoy or something you don't need to waste any more time fearing. Always try three times.

In the process of getting healthy, you're going to come face-to-face with fears you may have kept at bay for a long time. They will feel new to you but likely have just been buried. So it's best to identify and figure out how to manage them. The simple answer is (you guessed it) being uncomfortable. (Hang in there—the entire next chapter is about getting comfortable being uncomfortable.)

In the meantime, I'll share some actions you can take to help face your fears head-on using the tools you already have.

Do you fear success? How about the thoughts of not being worthy or deserving? You learned quite a bit about self-sabotage in Chapter Six. You know you're worthy and deserving of love and success, so you have to push out negative self-talk. Recognize your self-sabotage as a reaction to fear. What is standing between you and the life you want is your inability to navigate this fear. Take charge of your thoughts. Your negative self-talk and overthinking *What if...* are the only thoughts standing in your way.

Every time you experience a negative thought creeping in, kick it out. You can practice as you read this book. As you're reading some of these chapters, are you afraid I might be right? That you'll have to take responsibility? That's another fear, so write it down. When you read a sentence and your mind spits out the opposite negative feeling—stop, recognize it for what it is, and fix it. Change it to the positive. Retrain your brain.

It's time to act and start making life happen. You're afraid? Guess what—we all are. Do it anyway. Give yourself a chance to start feeling the rewards of success. Take one small step at a time. A great place to start is doing the homework in this book. Baby steps. Every single step will start building on each other. Small successes will be the beginning of your foundation for change. It will give you the strength to take more steps and start pushing out from under the what-ifs.

GRACE AND SUCCESS

I'll probably say this with every tool: leave room for grace. The reality is that we stumble. We think we have overcome a fear only to backtrack and shrink away from it sometime later. If you're thinking I have everything together and fear nothing, you're missing a big part of the message I am hoping to relay. I don't like hearing that practice makes perfect. I don't know what perfection is or even looks like.

We are human. Stumbles are opportunities to learn and grow. Sometimes you'll face a fear in three tries, sometimes it will take one try and you'll love it, sometimes you'll need much more practice. Give yourself as much grace as you would give your child, spouse, or anyone you love.

Make time to celebrate your successes. People who have hidden behind their fat armor for years tend to shy away from rewards and celebration. I find it interesting that this is one area we all tend to write off as no big deal. It's viewed as boasting or has the potential to draw attention we want to avoid.

Time to let go of that notion. You're doing hard work. You're making hard choices, all the time. Not just in this season but throughout your life. It's time to celebrate your efforts and results. Every single success is proof you can do this. Celebrate them. Fear is lost in victories. When you genuinely celebrate a victory, fear is not what you're feeling.

FREE: AUGUST 3, 2017

Happy birthday to me! Wow, I had no idea that he had arranged a day of zip-lining to celebrate my birthday. But those feelings of love and surprise were quickly taken over by fear. However, I had declared that it was time to start doing all the activities I'd only dreamt of from the couch and this was on top of my list. I was excited. I was full of fear, but I was choosing to control it rather than allowing it to let me back out.

Fear was no longer in control, though I'm not sure my legs, which were shaking uncontrollably, realized that. Standing on the platform, I was thinking that it just may take someone pushing me off. I just needed to lift my feet. It was so hard. The guides knew how to handle fears, which made me realize that many before me had likely been right there, not wanting to take that tiny step off the platform. Somehow that made me feel a little better, knowing they had done it and survived.

It took some self-talk. It took support and encouraging words. They were all very patient. My palms were sweaty and my heart was racing. I felt the fear pulsing through me. I was okay. I was facing my fear before I even took a step off the platform.

And then, I just lifted my feet and off I went. I was flying. I was so proud of myself. I did it. I faced my fear. I was free.

> **YOUR LESSON:**
> **Face your fears.**

FAT TO FREE ACTION PLAN

1. Write down any fears that are holding you back from losing weight. What are you worried about? Start your sentence off with "I am afraid that..."

2. Write a list of activities that scare you that you want to try in the next year, like riding a roller coaster, going down a slide, go-karting, rafting, or anything you could not do because your weight was a limitation. Or maybe there is something you have always wanted to do with your loved ones. It can be as simple as running with your kids or playing on the floor.

3. Write a list of all the blessings you're grateful for. This is excellent to refer to when you're scared, as it will replace the discomfort with good feelings. Add to this list every time you identify something new you're grateful for.

4. Pick one small fear you'd like to address within the next two weeks. Write out the fear and then a more positive outcome. For example, say you'd like to start making eye contact with others more often. The positive impact of pushing through that fear would be that you might make them smile or even meet some new friends.

Don't worry—you do not have to face your fears without some help to learn how to deal with all the discomfort you are feeling.

CHAPTER THIRTEEN: GETTING COMFORTABLE BEING UNCOMFORTABLE

FAT: APRIL 4, 2010

I want to tear the bandage off. I'm scared but at a point of belief that it has to hurt less and be easier than what I feel now. I want to live. I want to get off this couch.

STARTING SMALL

After the last chapter, you may already be feeling uncomfortable thinking about dredged-up fears. If that's the case, take a moment right now to note that you're okay. You're safe. You're in control.

Now think back: Were you ever taught how to navigate being uncomfortable? Discomfort is a temporary feeling, and if you push through, it will decrease. I've mentioned a few times already that much of this journey is going to be uncomfortable. In this chapter, you're going to learn how to get comfortable with those feelings.

Being fat puts you in a state of being uncomfortable often. I would go as far as betting that you spend most of your day that way. I did. Being uncomfortable is not going to go away, but you can learn how to navigate it.

You have to start small, so let's do a little exercise right now to give you an idea of what I'm talking about. Cross your arms in front of you—like so many of us do just out of habit—close your eyes, and sit still. Notice this feeling of comfort. Sit for one minute and then come back. Yes, put this book down and actually do it.

Welcome back. No big deal, right? Okay, now I want you to try it again, this time cross your arms the other way. This is even hard for some of us to do as it is out of our habitual way of doing it. Sit for one minute and observe how you feel.

This is an incredibly easy exercise to help you start to become comfortable with being uncomfortable. Baby steps.

The first result you should notice is that you survived! Observe that you're okay. I want you to do it again, but this time tell yourself, "I am going to be okay. No harm is going to come to me."

Immediately after you've experienced something uncomfortable, do something that brings you joy and makes you feel safe. Remember, you learned how to reward yourself earlier in the book. This is just another way of reprogramming your thoughts and actions with positive rewards rather than food.

Now the fears and discomfort you will face on your weight-loss journey are a taller order than folding your arms.

Here are some tips to help you push through when you're feeling uncomfortable.

◇ Notice the discomfort. Acknowledge it. Sit in it. Realize that you're okay.

After you've done this for a few minutes, switch to an activity you enjoy. Call a friend, go on a walk, listen to some music.

Don't skip the first part though. If you only try to bury the discomfort by switching activities without acknowledging how uncomfortable you are first, it will come back.

◇ Be grateful.

Gratitude leads to a positive outlook. When you're scared or uncomfortable, being grateful can replace the discomfort with good feelings and bring you joy. You can choose to do this either in the morning to kick off your day or while lying in bed at night.

Journal at least five items each day.

◇ Refocus your fear.

You can talk yourself through a difficult moment by reminding the fear that you have control and it doesn't. Let your fear know that you understand it has a place, but it doesn't get to rule your life.

Ask it questions like, "What's the worst thing that can happen?" Come up with the most ridiculous possible outcomes. They might even be humorous and allow you to laugh at your fears. That's an incredible feeling.

◇ Respect your fears and honor your courage.

Honor yourself when you have the courage to work through tough emotions and not allow fear to control you. Share your courage with a friend or your loved ones.

FAT TO FREE ACTION PLAN

Practice being uncomfortable to help build confidence. What do you fear that you have not told a friend? Write it down first and then share.

YOU GOT THIS

Change leaves all of us feeling off-balance sometimes. When life doesn't happen the way you want or expect, it leads to discomfort. Your response to change is key in your success. Ride it out and settle in, because life is always shifting, and you've got to grow and adapt. You have to learn to feel uncomfortable and still walk through it...or even sit through it.

You'll use this technique repeatedly and for the rest of your life. Learn to recognize that you're okay. Your fear will pass. Take a deep breath and say out loud, "I got this!"

Some fears and discomfort require more intense work. Here are some suggestions for tackling those.

◇ Learn from others.

Find someone who has experienced the same fear as you and ask how they managed it. Not only can you get some great tips, it also helps just to realize you're not alone.

getting comfortable being uncomfortable | 128

◇ Meditate.

Two years ago, you would never have found me meditating. I didn't understand the importance, and I thought it was too out there for me. Though I have a long way to go in learning how to meditate, I now practice every day at least once.

Each night, I go to sleep listening to a meditation track by Joseph Clough. He has many tracks that fall in line with the kind of feelings I am having or issues I like to tackle. Most of them are around 30 minutes, which is the minimum of self-care you should be doing each day.

These days, you can find plenty of apps and programs that make meditation easy and accessible. This practice is calming and helps ground me when I am feeling out of control, which is most often when life challenges are happening that throw off my plans or leave me feeling displaced. And let's be real—that is often. That is life.

◇ Educate yourself.

Books are a great way to learn more about yourself. Choose two books to read in two months that fall in line with the goals you are working on.

One of my favorite books is *Don't Sweat the Small Stuff...and It's All Small Stuff*. One chapter talks about how we should aim for the eye of the storm. In hurricanes, this refers to the center, where it's calm with clear skies, so people often think the storm has passed. In the eye, the storm swirls around you but you're safe.

Step out of the negative clouds, the high emotions, and any of the hype all around you. Live in the eye of the storm.

Does your work situation have a lot of stress that you and your coworkers spend a great deal of time talking about? Or maybe family events are filled with a bunch of drama? What would it look like if you took yourself out of the conversation?

To identify these types of scenarios, step back and ask if your actions are having any impact on the outcome. If they're not, step out of the chaos and into calm.

Set boundaries with others and let them know you do not want to participate. Careful—they will work hard to draw you back in, as you just put a spotlight on their behavior.

◇ Let go of control.

Are you aware of all the aspects of your life that you are giving energy to that you do not have control over? Write those out and identify the ones you are going to let go of. Work through your list.

Remember to revisit it because you may find yourself in new situations that need to be identified. Oftentimes the mere idea that we don't have control of a situation induces fear and discomfort.

The Serenity Prayer helps many people navigate through what they cannot control so they can become more grounded.

"God, grant me the serenity to accept the things I cannot change; courage to change the things I can; and the wisdom to know the difference."

◇ Center yourself.

Take a deep breath, go on a walk, ride a bike, exercise, and get refocused. Nature is proven to have a calming effect, so even just sitting in your backyard each day can be helpful. Get out of the storm of emotions surrounding whatever you're facing.

FAT TO FREE ACTION PLAN

Pick one item from the list you just wrote and make it happen. Write about what you chose and the experience you had.

Learning to appreciate discomfort doesn't have to be a single, grandiose action. Tomorrow, drive, bike, or walk a new route to work or to the store. You'll make it there just fine. Look around on your new route. Maybe you'll discover a new business or a beautiful home. It's a small action out of your normal routine and may provide a hint of discomfort. Embrace it. You'll be okay.

Next time, get fuel at a different station, wear a new outfit you've been holding on to, or throw on some bright lipstick. There are so many small tasks you can try that will be just slightly out of your comfort zone and allow you to practice your new skills.

Want to involve others? Take a coffee and tea order for your office mates. The deal is that everyone can have a drink, but they cannot have the one they ordered, including you. It will be different, but you may discover something new.

What you should note is that you can navigate through feeling uncomfortable. You may learn that you like a new drink or that your preference is different from what you thought. This is what will happen initially with most new experiences you fear.

Don't expect instant results. It will take time to develop this new skill. But don't overcomplicate the actions you need to take. This work is critical to putting your negative thoughts in perspective.

FREE: FEBRUARY 17, 2019

Last year [at our big gala event for work], I counted 32 people who hugged me but had never paid any attention to me before. Why now? Because my body is smaller? Does that make me more approachable? Last year, it annoyed me. It made me uncomfortable! This year, I celebrated it. I gave hugs to everyone. Last night felt good. I knew I looked good.

The people in this room have watched me transform over the last two years. I knew they would notice, and I knew there would be a buzz about it throughout the room. Uncomfortable! So I decided to make a joke out of it.

I stood tall and started my speech by saying that I knew they had one burning question on their minds: "Dang, girl, how did you lose all that weight?" It worked. They giggled and now they could just talk to me about it if they wanted.

YOUR LESSON:
Be comfortable being uncomfortable.

FAT TO FREE ACTION PLAN

1. Identify at least five activities you can do that will make you feel uncomfortable.

2. Decide when you will do them.

3. After you have done each one, come back to your journal and write what you experienced. Did you discover something new about yourself or others? Will you repeat the activity again? Did it stir up any unexpected emotions within you?

4. Did you reward your success? Return to your list of non-food rewards and update it.

Are you noticing any changes yet? Your efforts are far beyond the number on a scale, so keep your eyes open.

CHAPTER FOURTEEN: MORE THAN A NUMBER

FAT: AUGUST 24, 2013

Came out of the denial phase and accepted that not only am I fat, but I am also sick. I am killing myself. My denial has been to everyone else, because I've known it. You don't have painful feet, trouble with your eyes, Type 2 diabetes, huge clothes, double chins, and so many other symptoms without realizing this.

LET'S GET PHYSICAL

Do you remember taking a physical education class in school? PE, gym, conditioning, or maybe it was called something else for you—but definitely an awkward stage in life! Your body was developing, hormones were kicking in, and you were unsure if what was happening to your body was even normal.

I dreaded having to change into unflattering, uncomfortable unisex shorts and a t-shirt that always felt too small. We'd spend the class practicing some new activity. My coordination was nonexistent, which made physical education awkward. Dodgeball was the worst. I did find a great love for running at one point and was a member of the track and cross-country teams, but the rest of the class was misery.

As much as I dreaded the uniform, the once-a-month weigh-in was worse. Our weight was read out loud in front of everyone. You either heard something like "Way to go, you're healthy!" or a recommendation to eat healthier and exercise more. Even now, thinking about it makes my skin crawl. All my classmates judging me, my worth as a friend based on a number on the scale. The shame started early.

I wasn't even overweight then, but the scale was already defining my acceptance by others and whether I was cool or not. Classmates much larger than me were laughed at and shamed. I feared that would be me someday.

Today I have a whole new appreciation for that scale. I like to think of it as my compass, my guide. It navigates me in the right direction. Many people in my life who are not a part of my weight-loss program question why I weigh myself every day. I understand the conflict, because some believe that your weight is used to decide your worth. But by now, you realize that you're worthy and deserving of everything you want in life.

EMBRACE THE SCALE

Your weight is only telling you a story. Our bodies are amazing and speak to us often. The scale is just part of interpreting what your body is trying to tell you. If used as a proper tool, it's a window into what your body is doing or experiencing. It will tell you if you didn't get enough sleep. It will tell you if you ate a food that caused inflammation. With information like that, you can adapt your choices in real time.

Now of course it's also keeping your weight in check. Once you're healthy and you're living with the fact that you never want to go back to where you were, the single best tool to help is the scale. If you stop weighing in, it will be easy to convince yourself you're doing fine. You may feel your clothes get a little tighter or your fingers may seem puffy, but old habits of denial can return. Then fear can get the best of you and you won't want to get back on the scale.

It's a slippery slope that could land you right back where you started. Get on the scale, every day.

The great news is that you're not in school anymore. You don't need to compare your numbers to anyone else. Stay in your own lane. You get to determine (with your doctor) your ideal weight. Then you have to do the work to get there and stay there.

This is another time to be patient with yourself. Through this journey, you may stop losing weight, or you might go three steps forward and two steps back. When this happens, remember there are so many other successes you can observe and celebrate. Be kind to yourself and keep moving forward.

Don't forget that the scale is just one tool, one window sharing just one part of your body's story. Have you started to notice any other changes? Do any of these apply?

◇ Do your clothes fit differently?

◇ Is your eyesight better?

◇ Are aches and pains diminishing?

◇ Are you experiencing increased energy and confidence?

◇ Have you noticed your nails and skin are healthier?

◇ Are you fitting into smaller spaces?

◇ Are your shadow and reflections different?

◇ Have you noticed being less tolerant of negativity?

Recognize these changes and celebrate them.

By now, you have determined several rewards to celebrate completing your objectives and changing old habits. You're doing hard work, and these non-scale victories are just as fantastic as losing weight.

FREE: NOVEMBER 22, 2018

I did it. I wore my dream outfit! A white shirt tucked into jeans with a belt and boots. This journey has been about so much more than the scale. I even made it through a huge family Thanksgiving meal without eating any of the foods I knew would make me sick. I chose to fuel my body in a way that I knew I could still wear the outfit again tomorrow.

I think all the money I've been saving now that I am healthier is going to go toward shopping. It's kind of fun! No more tents for clothes. Oh, I'll have to go to Victoria's Secret. That scares the crap out of me, but I guess that means I have to do it.

YOUR LESSON:
Use a scale to listen to your body.

FAT TO FREE ACTION PLAN

If you don't have a scale yet, get one.

Write in your journal how it's going to be a helpful tool in your life to help you conquer one of your greatest challenges and then be instrumental in helping you never needing to climb this mountain again.

Get creative with how you are going to track your weight loss. I have seen elaborate charts on a wall, paper chains (remember the kind you use to make in elementary school out of construction paper?), or even marbles in a jar that represent each pound you want to lose.

Pick a time period and commit to tracking your weight.

Making mistakes is so often overrated. We all make them. Have you ever considered embracing them?

CHAPTER FIFTEEN: LEARNING FROM YOUR STUMBLES

FAT: SEPTEMBER 6, 2013

Holy heck. Chinese food for dinner. SO NOT WORTH IT!

September 23, 2013

So disappointed. I ate lots of junk this weekend. Two brownies, Cheetos, and a slice of pizza. But today is a new day...

HITTING A WALL

On a visit to see Sophie at college, I shared lunch with three wonderful ladies who were all at different stages of their weight-loss journeys. One was just starting—she was excited and feeling strong. One had been on the path for some time and was pleased with her success. She had lost over 120 pounds but then started struggling and put 20 back on. The third told us about her on-again/off-again story. She had lost

40 pounds and spent two days off insulin before self-sabotage kicked in. As a result, she regained the weight and was back on insulin.

Listening to their stories, I could hear the shame and judgment they attached to every past, current, and even future choice. But I get it, and I'm guessing you do too. It could be weight loss or some other life goal we just can't seem to reach. We all shame ourselves into believing we're not good enough and can't do it.

Over lunch, they all had questions about my journey. To my surprise, the issue we spent the most time on wasn't how I'd lost the weight. Instead they wondered...

"How did you climb over that wall I seem to run into over and over again?"

"How do you keep going?"

"How do you make it last?"

We all know how it goes. You get started, you lose some weight, you may even get a few pounds away from your goal, and then you end up going back to old ways. The story is typical: Life happened, stress levels were high, or you were simply at a restaurant with your favorite dessert. It started when you told yourself, "It's okay, I can have just one piece of cake."

Most of us know that moment. We're faced with a situation out of balance from our goals or our plan. We've felt that wall, looked up at it, and maybe even started to climb over it. And then we begin our fall backward with a choice. The situations may change, but the pattern is the same every time.

The choice. The guilt. The frustration. The disappointment.

We've gone back the way everyone in our life expected us to go. Their judgment was right; we were wrong. We start to justify to ourselves that it's easier to stay fat. After all, it's what everyone expected.

I can imagine you nodding in agreement. Please stop that!

Try this on instead: "It doesn't matter what others expect of me. I am going to continue on this journey and do what it takes to accomplish my goals."

NO ONE IS PERFECT

I spent years in counseling trying to figure out why I didn't have the life I wanted. Hundreds of hours and thousands of dollars later, I learned that what I wanted doesn't exist. I believed that everyone else had an easier life than me. I believed there was a secret I didn't have. Other people seemed to always be happy and, in my mind, they never faced any of the life challenges I had every day.

But the truth is, everyone has challenges, everyone falls. The difference is whether you choose to use those as excuses or lessons.

Similarly, these new friends I had lunch with (and many other people) assumed I never struggle anymore since I've lost weight. But in order to be successful in my weight loss, I needed to learn how to fall.

The word *cheat* brings along a trunk full of negative feelings. *Stumble* has far less stigma attached. A stumble is temporary, just a quick moment. This is how we should address challenges rather than letting them become defeating moments that set us back to square one. If you expect perfection, you're setting yourself up for additional failure.

You just have to start. No excuses. This practice is absolutely what has gotten me through. You'll definitely stumble, because food is everywhere and you're human. You have an addiction. Willpower only lasts so long, or (as mentioned previously) does it even exist?

But as you realize by now, you have complete control of how you respond.

Your life may include raising children, running a household, caring for elderly parents, and working at a job. Throw in some hobbies and friends and it's likely to feel hectic and busy much of the time.

One area I needed to focus on was learning to separate myself from any unnecessary craziness. Remember when I talked about finding the eye of the storm? Many times in my life there was a hurricane of emotions—mine and everyone else's—swirling around me. And once it started, it would find more and more garbage to throw into the disruption, increasing in size as it continued on its path.

Now I realize how often I was part of the storms destructive path, helping it grow, even for situations that were not my concern. What a mess. My family is full of high-drama people. With that in place, it is easy to react rather than sit back and listen and reflect before responding.

One time, my mom told us all she had a big announcement to make and none of us children could bring spouses, children, or cell phones. Well, this had the three of us all up in arms. We guessed that maybe she was leaving our dad or feared that she was sick.

By the day of the announcement, we were all exhausted from the storm we had created. Her news definitely made us speechless—it turns out we have a brother that she had given up for adoption many years ago and she had found him. Wow!

The point is, I had a choice: Instead of speculating and worrying and feeding into the fear, I could have told my brothers that we had no control over what Mom was going to tell us and that it would be best just to wait and see. Reminded them that she always had our best interests at heart. Suggested that we just wait and see. Stepped into the eye of the storm.

Through this journey of becoming free, I started to take charge of my response to others as well as my own emotional events. I removed myself from the drama surrounding me. Then I implemented a minimum three-day pause before responding to these emotional situations.

Where I've made the most progress practicing this is in my career as a nonprofit executive director. My weeks are filled with surprises and new challenges. Nonprofits are messy, as you are dealing with other people's time, money, and passions. There are many scenarios that can grow into high drama. And at times, you could find me right in the middle of it.

It could have been as simple as a debate between volunteers about what program should be implemented or more serious, such as discussing whether to let a volunteer go.

Over the years, I have improved my listening skills. Now when someone comes to me with a concern, I work to listen. And if it is a highly charged situation, I end the conversation by informing them I will get back to them. I take the time to research the situation and process the information. It also allows for everybody's emotions to settle. I get out of the chaos. Adding my emotionally charged opinion can wait until later. This is true in both my professional and personal lives.

This takes practice. If you're a knee-jerk responder like I've been all my life, it's hard not to respond in the moment. But almost anything can wait three days. This is another space you can practice getting comfortable being uncomfortable.

Here's another secret: When you pull yourself into the eye of the storm, it will eventually subside. You'll start to notice how often you unnecessarily engaged in situations or conflicts. This doesn't mean you can't be supportive, empathetic, or kind, it just means you don't give up your time, energy, or health for situations likely to resolve themselves regardless of your contribution. It sounds harsh, but it's not your problem.

LEARNING TO STUMBLE

Sophie was growing up, and it was time to start swimming lessons. Her prematurity had left her pigeon-toed and the doctors said to keep her active. She had done gymnastics, soccer, and dance, but she always loved the pool best.

We headed out for her first lesson with plans to go to her good friend's birthday party afterward. She was excited because she had chosen "the best Barbie doll ever" as a gift. The swim class was just Sophie and three other kids.

As we headed into the pool area, Sophie became a bit more clingy and worried about this new adventure. I encouraged her and told her how much fun she was going to have. There were three chairs for the parents; the children were asked to sit along the side and put their feet in the water.

But Sophie wouldn't do it. She wanted to sit in my lap and would not join the class. This frustrated and embarrassed me. I remember thinking, *Why did I spend all of this money for a lesson when she won't even sit on the side of the pool?*

My frustration turned to anger and I had no issue showing it. Then Sophie began to cry, which only fueled my anger. I demanded that she sit on the side of the pool with the other students, but she would not budge. At this point, I noticed the other parents staring at me in horror, which made my emotions go through the roof.

I plopped her down, grabbed her arm, and pulled her out of the pool area, letting her know that she was wasting my time and money and that there was nothing scary about sitting on the side of the pool.

It was one of those moments where you know you look a little unhinged but you can't stop. In my head, I was thinking I should stop, but the rage just kept building. When we were out of the pool area, I felt the eyes of the other moms on us.

I declared, "I am *not* taking you to your friend's party."

Her disappointment and sadness led her to say, "Okay, Mom. I'll go sit by the pool."

But then I said, "It's too late."

I was disgusted with myself and the scene I had just caused, which only led me to continue down the road of overreacting. I took it out on her, but my real frustration was with myself. We went home.

I cried that night. I felt terrible. Seeing her sadness and confusion was really hard on my heart. What was my tantrum about? I had messed up.

The next day, I apologized to Sophie for my behavior. I explained to her that it was more about me than her. I don't believe she understood that at the time, but her heart is so golden that she loved on me anyway. She listened as I explained that in the future if she was scared to do something that I wouldn't push her but rather let her decide when she was ready to try it. We also talked about my philosophy of trying things three times when scared.

Owning my actions, understanding why I had done it, and turning it into a learning opportunity was the easiest part for me. But I wasn't able to forgive myself or let go for a really long time.

We all stumble. Have you accepted that you will do this? Great. Now it's time to learn how to do it gracefully.

1. Own it.

    Don't let regret, guilt, or shame have any of your time or energy. Those are dark emotions that no longer serve you.

    You made a choice. Own it and learn from it. Every choice gives you the opportunity to take credit for creating your own life.

    Owning your life is powerful, and when you realize that, you'll focus on making decisions that create the life you want instead of blaming everything and everyone else. (Hernandez)

2. Understand why.

    There's a difference between seeking to understand and coming up with excuses. You need to identify what led you down this road. Take time to analyze the situation, name the emotions, and recall what was going on before you made the decision.

For example, if you ate junk food late at night, ask yourself whether you were bored, anxious, or something else. When you can recognize your situation, you'll know better how to respond to the actions.

This is not an opportunity to whine about life happening; it's a chance to pinpoint the feelings you experienced because life happened.

3. Forgive yourself.

Say it out loud. Say something like "I am not going to carry any shame or guilt beyond this moment because of my choices. Instead, I am going to forgive myself and turn this into an opportunity to learn. I am worthy of forgiveness."

You deserve the same kindness and forgiveness you would offer any of your friends and loved ones. Take the time to look at yourself in the mirror and apologize for not taking care of your body. If you harmed a friend or family member, you would apologize, right?

4. Let it go.

It is time to move on from your stumble. You won't do yourself any good sitting around and wallowing in decisions you already made. Remember, this is about action and changing your life. Let it go and move forward.

5. Turn it into opportunity.

Be proactive and identify what can be fixed. What was your trigger?

Assess the situation and ask yourself fact-finding questions so you can adjust as necessary next time. Did you use your tools? If not, why? Do you need to update your list of safeguards, rewards, or experiences to be more appealing? Do you need to better prepare for a new situation you're facing?

Review your response and adjust it for a better outcome.

FAT TO FREE ACTION PLAN

1. Write down what you were feeling at a time when you stumbled on your weight-loss journey. Get into detail about what happened and how you reacted.

   • Did you realize you were choosing to stuff your emotions?

   • What kind of feelings were you experiencing from beginning to the end, and even now?

   • Have you forgiven yourself, and did it take more than just saying it and releasing it?

2. If you are still hanging on to guilt, write about why that might be. Be sure to include what you need to do to let it go and move on.

3. Develop your plan for next time. Be specific.

No matter what you've done, there's always hope for the future. This is an opportunity to learn from that experience. It's one time you have full control to adjust and adapt. The past is the past. The only real moment is right now. It's up to you to make choices in this moment that leave you feeling happy and positive.

And you know what? When you get up, you'll absolutely stumble again. But once you've learned how to fall, each time it becomes shorter and getting up becomes easier. The lessons you learn become additional tools you can use.

Here are some examples of actions to try when you stumble.

◊ STOP IT. (Simple but powerful!) Put the food down and walk away. Remove the food temptations from your home. Choose to find a different way to respond to your emotions.

◊ Increase your water intake. Your body is inflamed from the junk food, and you need to flush it out.

◊ Stay accountable. If you're following a weight-loss program that requires tracking food, don't skip it if you overeat or eat something bad. Record everything. You need to see exactly what you did and the impact on the scale. If you lie to your food log, you're only lying to yourself.

◊ Consider why you stumbled and adjust your safeguards if needed.

◊ Review your affirmations: "I am worthy!" (This tool is coming up next.)

◊ Remember the sickness and loss you've witnessed and experienced. Remember why you're making new choices.

◊ By this point, you should be surrounded by reminders of your why. Put on a piece of clothing that reminds you how far you've come.

◇ Look in the mirror and name three non-scale victories you're enjoying because of your positive choices and lifestyle changes.

◇ Choose health! Create an action plan, including measurable objectives. Get back on track immediately.

◇ You should be your loudest cheerleader, and you can start by giving yourself a good talking to.

FREE: FEBRUARY 23, 2020

It's uncomfortable that even as I am writing my book, I'm still learning and unpacking. As I write that, I'm laughing at myself. Duh, life challenges don't go away.

Tonight I'm dealing with regrets and the losses that are a direct result of my choices to remain fat and hide from life. Old habits want to creep back in. It would be so easy to order takeout. Damn, our society has made it so easy to eat large amounts of food without anyone else knowing. Pie. Pizza. Burgers. Fries. All of it dancing in my head.

I'm sad. I'm crying. I'm feeling it. Fighting off the desire to stuff away my pain. Oh crap, my old habits still get me. How many times did I look in the pantry tonight? Thank goodness I don't have any junk in the house. I've got to let this pain out so there's nothing to stuff. Shower, sleep, and start again.

FAT TO FREE ACTION PLAN

What happens when your old habits get the best of you? What is your plan if you stumble? Write a list of what will work best for you. When you stumble, pull out this list and you'll know exactly how to react in a positive way that stays in line with your goals. Then getting back on track will be so much easier.

CHAPTER SIXTEEN: TALKING TO YOURSELF

FAT: DECEMBER 11, 2015

I feel stupid. I feel empty. I am lonely. Something is wrong with me. I'm starting to believe that this is just the life I was destined to have. I'm trying to express myself and share my needs. I hear the words come out of my mouth, but they don't lead to understanding or change. Why can't I get this right?

WHAT THEY DIDN'T KNOW

Each year, the nonprofit organization I work for hosts a fundraising event in a small, prosperous town. As the executive director, I have to stand up in front of more than 500 prominent guests and speak. This formal event requires dress shopping each year, and in the spirit of being uncomfortable, I'd take the opportunity to judge myself before others judged me.

I'd always announce how had to go "muumuu shopping." This was my way of deflecting my absolute discomfort with the entire process. I'd have to spend eight hours in a formal dress that felt like a tent and standing on my feet, which by the end of the night hurt so bad that I could barely walk. And I'd have to smile the whole way through.

I had a routine to get through the night. The evening always starts with a schmoozing cocktail hour. I'd get dressed up and make an appearance, so people knew I was around. Then I'd excuse myself to go practice my speech. But while I practiced, I'd also order room service and eat to calm my nerves.

The hotel staff knew my routine—one meal during the event and another waiting for me at the end of the night. If I ever mentioned nerves, everyone suggested I do a shot of alcohol. I'd always decline, and they would be impressed that I could go on stage without that boost of courage. They had no idea that food was all I needed.

Through eating, I buried my shame of being fat deep enough so I could return to the ballroom for the main event. The next challenge was to map out how to get to the stage. You see, 500 people in a room means chairs were back-to-back. To avoid embarrassment, I had to plan out a path where I could squeeze through the aisles. It was never easy. By this time, my toes were purple and my legs hurt from my ankles up to my butt. But I kept smiling and schmoozing. I kept going, all while my mind was reeling with fear, guilt, shame, and disgust.

Oddly enough, people always told me how great I did. At the end of the night, I'd go back to my room, sit in the bathtub with cold water running on my feet, take large quantities of pain relievers, and (of course) eat again.

I doubt anyone else at the event had any idea how torturous this experience was for me. Some might even wonder how on earth I pulled off a professional career while filled with such sadness, anguish, and despair.

I've been blessed with two main things through this entire journey—hope and the certainty in my soul that I had something to offer others. For a long time, I just wasn't sure exactly what that was or how I'd share it with the world.

TALKING AND LISTENING

Affirmation is another buzzword I heard when I started this journey. At first, I responded with monumental eye rolls and disregarded the message. It was so easy to dismiss. What good can talking to yourself do?

Let me tell you, it can do a lot of good.

But there's one catch: What you say must be positive. And you have to be willing to listen. In fact, I encourage you to talk to yourself every day.

End any negative self-talk. This includes thoughts when someone tells you that you look nice or when your boss gives you a compliment. Maybe your spouse adores you and you make comments to put yourself down rather than saying thank you. If you don't stand up for and believe in yourself, you can't expect anyone else to either. Keep them positive; avoid using words like "not" or "nothing." This is about getting the negative thoughts out.

Affirmations are positive declarations to help you overcome self-sabotaging and negative thoughts. Your affirmations should be short statements in the present tense, starting with "I am" or "I choose." Be specific and include one strong word or emotion that resonates with you. For example, "I will lose and keep off the weight" or "I will treat myself with self-respect."

They can decrease stress levels and minimize negative thoughts. The more you become conscious of your thoughts—the negative things your brain is telling you—the more you can ensure they are positive and the better your life can be.

Benefits to speaking affirmations aloud daily include the following:

◇ Boosting your problem-solving skills

◇ Helping you perform better under pressure

◇ Helping you remember what you want in life

◇ Reconnecting with feelings of gratitude

◇ Focusing your perspective on the good aspects of life

When I started using affirmations, I was told to simply write them down at first, even if I didn't feel they were true. I needed to practice and give it time to work. So basically, I faked it for a long time. I had to trust the process and stop overthinking, so I went for it. Fake it till you make it, right?

At first, I felt odd and uncomfortable. I stayed the course and every morning looked in the mirror and said my affirmations. Within just a couple of weeks, I started to notice other people's negativity to the point that it would bother me. It was not comfortable to be around.

My other observation was that I felt joy and had a skip in my step. Each day became a bit brighter. And then one day, about six weeks into my affirmations, I noted that

I said the affirmations a bit differently, with more confidence. I felt good. I felt strong. I felt positive.

These may be difficult to put in writing. Or you may already have some that jump to mind. Write your affirmations even if you don't believe them just yet. You will. Write them if you're scared or uncomfortable—you can face that fear. You may feel extremely vulnerable. That's okay.

My affirmations are personal, and only recently have I been able to share them without emotions taking over. When I started using them, I had a level of shame associated with saying them. I did not feel worthy to say them to myself, much less to anyone else. I was still holding on to many regrets that I had associated with being a single mom, my failed marriage, and by this point, another failing relationship. I feared my own judgment for even saying the words, and also judgment from others.

How on earth could anyone love me after the life I had lived and the choices I made?

The emotion comes from the path I have been on since I wrote them. There is something powerful about writing affirmations. I went from thinking they were just a fake practice exercise to now believing without a doubt that I am worthy and proud of the woman I have become.

Once you've written your affirmations, practice them while looking in the mirror. Make this part of your morning routine. Look yourself in the eyes and say each one slowly and clearly several times. Don't question it, don't fight it, just do it. It doesn't matter if you feel stupid—this is for your ears only. Take your time, be reflective, and consider what you're saying to yourself.

Another great tip is to say your affirmations while standing in the Superman pose. Stand tall with your head tilted up and your hands on your hips. It is a confident pose. Try it. It does make a difference. Maybe because it forces you to slow down and think about what you are saying. Afterward, you will walk out of your bathroom feeling ready for the day.

I still speak at that fundraising event every year, but now it's much different. Don't get me wrong—I'm still nervous. But shopping for a dress has become fun. My feet still hurt (because heels), but now I have two pairs of shoes to get me through the evening, and I make sure they fit correctly ahead of time.

When I sneak away to review my speech, instead of eating, I take a deep breath, get in my Superman pose, and say my affirmations. This builds up my confidence and reminds me that everyone in the audience is there for the same reason.

The evening is much more enjoyable when I'm not worrying about anyone knowing how much I eat, wondering who's judging me because of how I look, or thinking that no one is listening to my speech. More importantly, now I know that was never the case—it was all my negative self-talk. Even if someone is judging me for any reason, I know it's not my problem, it's theirs.

I no longer need to map out a pathway or worry about getting stuck between chairs in the middle of the room. Oh, I still get stuck. Who wouldn't with 500 people? But now I just look people in the eye, smile, and say, "Excuse me."

Practice your affirmation statements every day. Use them at times that are stressful or when you're being triggered and want to eat through a scenario. Practice them until they become reality and you truly believe every word you're telling yourself.

FREE: OCTOBER 18, 2017

I am good enough. I am intelligent. I am worthy of love and respect. I got this. I am Elizabeth.

YOUR LESSON:
Learn to use affirmations.

FAT TO FREE ACTION PLAN

1. Write down some affirmations.

2. Say them out loud.

3. Choose an activity from your reward list and celebrate!

After all this hard work, you deserve some self-care. Read on to learn many different ways that you can do that for yourself.

CHAPTER SEVENTEEN: MORE THAN A SPA DAY

FAT: APRIL 4, 2010

Time to take care of myself.

Nutrition: Cook at home, eat out no more than one time per week, drink no more than 6 pops a week.

Exercise: At least 30 minutes, 4 times per week

Financial: Find a financial planner.

Work: Change schedule to 8 a.m.–4 p.m., take breaks.

WHAT IS SELF-CARE?

My mom, always a loving care provider, inspired me to keep going and complimented me for all I was doing. If anyone in my life saw even a bit of my misery, it was her. She wanted me to find my way out but was unsure how to help. At the same time, she was the last person I was going to listen to. Isn't that odd? Our parents should be a rock in our world, but we also need to figure out how hard life is on our own.

While I was a single parent, going to school full time and working full time, my mom worried. She would ask what I was doing to care for myself, and my standard response was always, "I'm getting my nails done."

Self-care is another buzzword we throw around. What we often don't understand is that it's so much more than getting your hair and nails done. Self-care goes far beyond a few minutes of pampering yourself. Don't get me wrong, it's a great step, but just one of six areas you'll need to address at some point. When you list your daily objectives, ensure you're including some level of self-care from each of these categories:

- ◇ Physical
- ◇ Emotional
- ◇ Mental
- ◇ Spiritual
- ◇ Practical
- ◇ Social

PHYSICAL SELF-CARE

Physical self-care includes any activity you do to improve the well-being of your body. You've made it this far in the book, so you should already be taking measures to care for your physical self. Ending your emotional eating is key to this process, combined with learning how to fuel your body. Other activities you should focus on for your physical well-being include sleep, hydration, and physical movement.

Note that I didn't say *exercise*. That word scares so many. You get to decide how you'll move your body. It can be anything, like taking walks, riding bikes, or lifting weights. Any movement that feels good for your body will do, just move it.

EMOTIONAL SELF-CARE

Emotional care is anything to help you connect, process, and reflect. This is a critical piece in addressing your emotional eating.

Have you ever invested in counseling? I did, but I didn't utilize it the way I should have. It became a crutch, a bitch session, more than an outside, professional perspective to help me process and reflect. I absolutely learned lessons and credit my counselor for helping me overcome some major life challenges, but it's not meant to be a substitute for doing the real work. Get in. Get the lesson. Practice it.

But maybe counseling is not for you. No problem, there are many other ways to practice emotional self-care. My favorites are writing and art. Have you seen adult coloring books? Don't judge. Buy one and some nice markers or pencils. Find a comfortable spot. Put on some music. Make sure any children and pets are cared for, and block out some time to color. You'll be surprised how just 30 minutes a day can help you get out of chaos and into the eye of the storm.

Meditate. Dance. Garden. Whatever you need to do. Dedicate time to connect with yourself. Check in to ensure you're staying true to your needs and objectives.

MENTAL SELF-CARE

Caring for your mental health includes any action that will stimulate your mind and intellect. I love this one. Learning new information lights me up, keeps boredom and overthinking at bay. (And we all know what most of us do when we're bored.)

Activities for your mental self-care include reading (or listening to) a book. Find a new podcast, do a puzzle, learn a new game like chess or backgammon, play cards. These are also excellent activities to do with your children or loved ones. Sophie and I have a tradition to buy a new puzzle each Christmas and do it together. I still need to learn chess but I have fond memories of playing backgammon and cards with my grandmother, Pauve, and my mom.

Find a stimulating activity you like, and make sure it's on your list of rewarding experiences you'll use instead of food.

SPIRITUAL SELF-CARE

Spiritual care includes activities that make you think bigger than yourself. This doesn't have to have a religious affiliation, but for many it does. Consider meditating, practicing yoga, dedicating time for reflection, going to church, or getting out in nature.

Do you have a place of peace, somewhere you can sit and absorb the beauty around you? One of my most reenergizing and spiritual times is when I'm sitting by the water. It doesn't matter if it's a river, lake, or ocean. The calm and connection I feel centers and relaxes me at a level I'm rarely able to capture in any other setting.

It's important to find calm and appreciate that there is a world beyond you. This is about looking beyond the bubble you focus on day in and day out. It's easy to become overwhelmed. This time is a reset button. It will give you direction and strength to help you move forward on your journey.

PRACTICAL SELF-CARE

Practical self-care is practicing tasks in the current moment in order to prevent future stressful situations. If you're a planner like me, this doesn't take much effort. Actions include tasks like creating a budget and managing your money, developing new professional skills, or even decluttering your house.

All these activities will help prevent future stress from unexpected circumstances. Decluttering your house can also remove an excuse many of us use: hiding. If I had to put clutter away, clean out closets, or reorganize drawers, I didn't have to face fears or join activities that made me uncomfortable. Once you end your toxic relationship with food, you're not going to want to be stuck at home!

It can be a chore to get started, but make time to declutter now so that when the weekends roll around you can get out and have some fun.

Take care of essential tasks as needed. Pay your bills. Maintain your car. Clean out the closets. These actions tell the world that you care about your life and that you make yourself a priority.

SOCIAL SELF-CARE

Social activities allow you to nurture and deepen relationships with people in your life. If you've been hiding from the world for much of your life, this might feel challenging. Trust me, I know. I was the queen of excuses. I routinely accepted social invitations but then didn't go. I did this over and over until everyone stopped asking. I couldn't overcome the anxiety or negative feelings. But as events were going on while I hid at home, I felt guilty and usually ate my way through those emotions.

Good news: To address your social self-care, you don't actually have to go out or accept all those invitations if you don't want to. Ease into it, and your opinion of social gatherings will likely change as you continue. Until you're ready though, pick up the phone and call a friend, your parents, or a family member just to say hello and that you love them.

Time is the greatest gift you can give anyone, including yourself. It can be over the phone, on a video chat, over coffee, or during a night out when you're ready. (Social media comments don't count!) Connect and build your relationships; they will only make you stronger.

Here are some other ideas to help you get started.

◊ Go to the library.

◊ Spend time outdoors.

◊ Write a letter.

◊ Watch the sun rise or set.

◊ Download a meditation app and try it out.

◊ Declutter a spot in the house.

◇ Wear an outfit that makes you feel good.

◇ Pay it forward.

◇ Read a book.

◇ Edit your social media followers.

◇ Go for a drive.

◇ Start a budget.

◇ Stretch for 20 minutes.

◇ Close yourself in a room to color, meditate, or listen to a podcast.

◇ Look at the stars.

◇ Have a 30-second dance party.

◇ Do something crafty.

◇ Take a walk somewhere new.

FREE: DECEMBER 8, 2019

Wow, that was a great weekend filled with friends. I worked around the house and even went on several dates. Who would have guessed that at 49 years old, I'd be back out trying to find that someone special to share my life with? Not me! Going out to meet someone who you've only texted with or seen pictures of online is definitely out of my comfort zone.

But wait—they listened to me. Like, genuinely took interest and asked follow-up questions about me. And even better, I answered from my heart. I was authentically myself. Not only did they listen, they also wanted to spend more time with me. I guess it's time to embrace the fact that I'm a pretty cool chick who has a great deal to offer. Now I just have to find a guy who I feel the same way about.

YOUR LESSON:
Practice all six areas of self-care.

FAT TO FREE ACTION PLAN

1. Write out what you'll do to address your self-care in each area.

    ◆ Emotional

    ◆ Mental

    ◆ Physical

    ◆ Practical

    ◆ Social

    ◆ Spiritual

2. Set specific goals for how and when you will do these activities.

Your body and mind are not the only changes that are going to come with this process. Experiencing the impact on your life is one of the best parts of this journey.

CHAPTER EIGHTEEN: LIFE AFTER WEIGHT LOSS

FAT: NOVEMBER 17, 2013

Weight logged for the day: 225.5 lbs. Holy cow! Wow, that's a first! Love it!

CHALLENGES AND VICTORIES

Extreme weight loss comes with new challenges, but they're nothing compared to what you've been doing. Let's get real for a minute. This journey has not been all roses and happiness. Significantly altering your body composition in this way is absolutely a blessing, but there are also bumps, and they don't all end when you reach your goal weight.

It's uncomfortable recognizing how you saw yourself and adjusting as you get to know your new self. It's emotional and can cause you to feel unsure where you fit in now. Remember that change can leave you feeling displaced, but it can help to get comfortable with being uncomfortable. It's an imperative tool you'll use for your entire life. It also helps to know what you can expect so you're not caught completely off guard. Set yourself up for success; the last thing you need is more emotions to trigger you.

For me, losing 100 pounds also brought me a list of victories completely unrelated to the number on the scale. These started early and continue to this day. I have plenty of successes to celebrate, and though they seem minor, there were challenges as well that should be shared.

The reason it's important for me to share them is to help others who fear what will be and use that as an excuse to stop moving forward. By reading what I've been through, you'll know some of what to expect, which will hopefully dissipate some of your fear and give you some milestones to look forward to.

"JUST MUSH IT"

The changes in my body were shocking and even painful. When Sophie was growing up and would fall or bump into something, causing tears, my go-to line was, "Mush it." I wanted her to get over the pain quickly and be tough. If she bumped into the corner of a table, I'd tell her to rub her calf, just massage out the pain. I had no idea what I was asking of her when I'd say, "You're okay. Mush it— that will help." How wrong I was.

One day, I was putting away dishes in the kitchen. I turned and knocked my shin on the corner of the dishwasher. I immediately heard in my head and all around me, *MUSH IT!* Ouch! You probably already know what I discovered. Not only was it bad advice, many people—especially kids— don't have a layer of fat protecting their bones.

Don't tell your kids, or anyone, to "Mush it." It hurts! Sophie and my bonus children, Katie and Kenny, were excited to know they would never hear me say that again.

My bones had been covered with fat for a long time. As that fat melted away, it physically hurt to be touched. It took weeks to get used to sitting on my tailbone. Sleeping on my side hurt. My hips needed time adjust to the loss. My whole body hurt, which also led to discomfort during sex. (Hopefully, you're in a good relationship and the two of you will figure it out.) The physical pain was surprising but also temporary.

The good news is that all the adjustments you'll experience are manageable.

YOUR *PRETTY WOMAN* MOMENT

When you've lived a life shopping in the clothing section of a full-service grocery store, walking through the mall can be intimidating. I started by going to the Gap with my daughter, because I could pretend I was just there to support her. I saw some sizes that might fit and grabbed a few items, then soon realized I could take my pick of outfits I liked.

At first, I stuck to ones that were not out of my comfort zone and would feel joy when they would easily slip over my head. I'd look in the mirror and think, *Dang, girl, you are looking good!*

As my confidence grew, I went out and chose items that in the past I could only imagine wearing, like shorter shorts or shirts that come off the shoulders. I grabbed them all and had so much fun trying them on. I took so many pictures. I cried happy tears. I didn't have to resort to whatever would just fit around my wide body. I could actually start figuring out my style.

This was a first step but certainly not the end of my fear. As I continued to shrink, I was excited to shop, but the fear in my head got the best of me several times. I'd be in a store looking around and out of habit I would go right to the women's sizes, where the clothes were now much too large for me. Regardless, my shopping habit before weight loss was never about style or being proud. It was about covering up, usually with dark colors so I wouldn't draw attention.

As your body shrinks and you discover you can shop in any store, you may become anxious. Asking for help may seem hard, but it will be worth it. You'll find out that sales-people love when you ask for help, because it pulls them away from having to fold sweaters! Tell them your story and they'll likely treat you like Julia Roberts in *Pretty Woman*. Which, by the way, you deserve! (Just don't let this cause a bigger problem for your bank account.)

Once you've lost a significant amount of weight, get rid of clothes that no longer fit. Your fat self will want to tuck them away...just in case. No more backup plans. You now have the tools to keep you from going backward. Clothes are a financial investment, so by getting rid of them you're also getting rid of that way out. In addition, you make the statement: "I am done with these clothes and they no longer serve any purpose for me." Then buy new ones that you love and celebrate your new body.

An excellent way to handle this practically and financially is by thrift shopping. When losing a great deal of weight, you'll go through several sizes quickly. Donate your old clothes, then pick up a few key items to get you through the next few weeks. Repeat until you hit your goal weight.

If you've also done some practical self-care and worked on your budget, save a little for your *Pretty Woman* moment as a reward.

Mostly, don't wait too long. Don't listen to any negative internal voice saying, "You don't deserve this" or "What if you gain the weight back?" At every step, you've got to push through the fear and not let it in. Truly believe that you're not going to gain your weight back this time because you're taking steps to fuel your body and stop using food as comfort and entertainment.

FOR THE LADIES

Bras? Well, that's another story. When I used to walk by specialty bra stores, I would run the other way. When I finally went into one, the experience wasn't nearly as bad as I'd worked up in my head. (Isn't that the truth for just about everything?)

At first, I avoided eye contact. I looked around at all the varieties, sizes, and options. Then the store associate helped me get started. I even documented the event on social media! The dressing room was pink, with a plush chair, antique hooks, and mirrors on the wall. My name was posted on the door. Not just a typical department store cubicle. I posted a picture of the beautiful dressing room and said, "Guess what I'm finally doing!" Why wouldn't I celebrate? This was a big deal.

My kind saleslady asked me about my weight loss and did not get upset when I wanted to try on almost a dozen bras. She was patient and helped soothe some of my anxiety.

All that and I still didn't enjoy it though. I am pretty sure I tried on every style of bra they had. They were all uncomfortable and exposed me in ways I wasn't used to.

I wanted to run, but I pushed through. I had to do this. I was uncomfortable, but I was okay. I was determined to find a bra I liked. I became increasingly discouraged and began closely looking at my body in the mirror. *Look at all that extra skin.* All my fears and negative voices were screaming, "RUN!" I even cried a little bit.

Finally, one bra I liked felt comfortable. But wait, it was still a "big" size. I stood in the dressing room feeling defeated and still fat.

So you should expect that trying new things will be difficult, but you must push through and avoid eating your emotions. Through this torturous bra-buying experience, I learned that I am not defined by the numbers and letters on the tag. I am defined by walking into that store and battling fear. I am defined by being uncomfortable and realizing that I don't need food to comfort myself.

FACING YOUR REFLECTION

It's unsettling to no longer recognize yourself. Sometimes you look in the mirror and you still see your fat self. Other times, you walk by a window and are startled at your reflection. *Who is that?* I remember one time being thrilled by my shadow being so small, but it still didn't quite register how it was connected to my physical self.

Your mind will want to pull you back to old ways, so you have to continue to embrace your new body. You may find yourself checking a mirror to confirm that you didn't get fat again. You have to get your brain to catch up with the changes. As odd as it sounds, checking yourself out in the mirror every day for at least 10 minutes will help. It's time for you to accept and love your new body. As you do this, repeat your affirmations (even if you still don't believe them). It works.

One day, you'll be walking down the street and see your reflection, but rather than be startled you'll smile and think, *Wow, that's me and I don't need to hide.* It's a great feeling.

INTIMACY AND RELATIONSHIPS

Several exciting changes happened in my romantic relationship as a result of weight loss. Our hands felt better entwined, our cuddles were closer, he could carry me, I could wear his clothes, and my sex drive was much higher. We started getting more active and working toward common goals rather than letting life pass us by.

Weekends turned into productive and fun adventures instead of arguments and chores. We enjoyed walking, bike riding, zip-lining, paddleboarding, canoeing, and boating. One of my favorite activities was when we ventured off to hike and find some hot springs. My guy bought me a HydraPak, and it felt good to be able to get out and have fun the way we had always talked about.

That was all good, but it's not the only characteristic that makes a relationship sustainable. Our 10 years together had been filled with mistakes and hurt. Neither of us came to the table being our true selves, and that led to a relationship full of blame, control, judgment, manipulation, guilt, and separation.

The love we shared in the beginning did appear on and off through the years when we tried to get back to all the dreams and goals we had planned. We were raising our kids together and oftentimes, as many relationships do, we would find ourselves with little left to give to each other. Our wounds were far deeper than what newfound confidence, energy, and joy could fix at that time. So we split up.

I was scared to be myself with anyone new because what if they didn't love me? Even more complicated was that I had no idea who I was. In all my efforts to be loved, not only was I lonely, I was also missing the vulnerable, loving relationship that I so desperately desired.

My eyes were opened to all of this on my journey. It was incredibly freeing to stop trying to be what I thought everyone else wanted me to be (which was different for each person in my life) and start showing everyone the real me. It's a big moment when you admit you have no idea who you are. But I've had fun figuring it out.

It's hard to explain the relief that comes with admitting your truth and accepting the outcome for whatever it may be. When you work to try to make someone respond the way you want rather than being your real self and allowing them to do the same, it leads to a lot of heartache and a feeling of never being heard. It was exhausting always working to try to feel love by saying what you thought that person wanted to hear.

An example would be when a loved one would ask me, "Do you want to go to the movies tonight?" I'd reply, "I would love to." Inside thinking how much I would rather take a walk, work in the garden, or even pull up a movie on the television rather than go out. This was beyond just making a sacrifice every now and then. This was a consistent choice of answering with what I believed they wanted to hear. The correct way would have been to say no thank you and offer up some other suggestions, with the result likely being some kind of compromise that resulted in a nice evening.

I wanted to be loved. I didn't want to lose my relationship. But all I did was push people away. I had to accept the fact that I never had control. I had tolerance and, at some levels, even the love I desired.

The problem is that when you're not being yourself in relationships, you exhaust your partner, and they'll eventually say, "I've had enough." It doesn't matter how much they loved you in the beginning or what commitment they made if it was never really "you" to begin with.

To survive this dramatic change, you must communicate frequently and effectively with your partner. Be vulnerable. Be you. Even though you have been hiding for years and want to discover your genuine self, you need to consider their feelings through this.

You're now on a journey of discovering who you truly are, and that includes learning how to be your best self with your loved ones, friends, and even family. This will have an impact on your relationships—some may flourish, but others may end.

Will people treat you differently once you've lost weight? Yes. And you'll wonder if it's because of you or because of them. My guess is a little bit of both. Others will pay more attention to you. They will look you in the eyes, greet you, and even help you in the grocery store. You may notice that service is better and casual conversation happens more often at restaurants and on airplanes.

The lie we tell ourselves is that the fat is protecting us. But it's not.

Vulnerability is uncomfortable regardless of whether you are overweight. But if you want to finally live a life true to yourself, you must experience this. You're doing a great deal of healing and discovering the new you, but you also have to determine how to share that with others.

Finding your voice and speaking up may feel uncomfortable at first, but as time goes on, you'll gain strength. This step in the process is hard because it requires you to address many emotions and insecurities that you've numbed for years with food. Using the tools in this book to navigate those emotions without food will help you move toward healing and loving yourself. That's so freeing!

GRIEVING THE LOSS OF FOOD

It may sound ridiculous to grieve over what you eat, but think about it: Food has played a major role in your life. It provided comfort. It filled time when you were bored. It entertained you. It celebrated with you. Now food will no longer fill those roles. That means you must change how you spend time with your loved ones and deal with these other situations in a different way.

Once you've lost the weight, you may be tempted to fall back to rewarding yourself with food because you worked so hard. You'll have to decide if you're going to let food continue to play any of these roles and, if so, what it will look like. Regardless, this journey changes your life, and you should prepare for some feelings of loss.

FAT TO FREE ACTION PLAN

These changes don't mean you have to also lose connections or skip all celebrations. Write about one of your favorite occasions. This could be family dinners, barbecues, camping, holidays, birthdays, lunches with friends, nights out with the girls, or graduations.

Write about the details that make you smile and bring you joy when reminiscing about the event. Next time you attend one of these events, carry these positive memories in your heart. The experience is what matters, the time spent together.

MAKING MEMORIES

We tend to think that food must be present at every event or social gathering because that's a habit. It's what society tells us to do. It's what social media convinces us we need for a good time. But it also comes back to food being used for comfort and entertainment instead of fuel.

Change your thinking and focus your time on the people and the activities rather than the meals. Here are some tips to get you started.

◊ Take charge of event planning so that you can make sure the schedule and activities are in line with your goals.

◊ Share your goals with others and ask for their support.

◊ Plan experiences, not meals.

◊ Before date night, talk to your significant other and come up with a list of new activities the two of you can go do together. Figure out other ways you can express and share love ways that don't involve food.

◊ At any function, if you're struggling, walk around to each person and learn one new story about them. It keeps you busy while you also build new connections.

COUNTING YOUR BLESSINGS

All the experiences I've described in this chapter may cause fear and possibly surprise, but each one can also be a celebration of your new lease on life. Sure, there will be challenges, but as you've learned, there will also be endless blessings.

Imagine you're already there...

◊ Your grocery bills are lower.

◊ Your energy is through the roof.

◊ You have stopped watching and started doing.

◊ Your confidence has increased.

◊ Your health has improved.

◊ You've increased your life expectancy and decreased your medical bills.

◊ Your skin looks better, and your hair feels healthier.

◊ You fit into smaller spaces.

◊ You lock eyes and smile with more people.

◊ You don't need a seatbelt extender.

◊ Your rings fit.

◊ You enjoy a piggyback ride.

◊ You no longer think about food all the time or wonder if you're the fattest person in the room.

◊ You sit on the floor with your children and get back up unassisted.

◊ You run.

◊ You bend over.

- You don't sweat from walking to get the mail.
- You're not out of breath going up the stairs.
- You tie your shoes.
- You wear a belt.
- Your sight is improved.
- You don't worry about breaking a chair.
- You don't hide your body.
- You don't flinch when you're touched.
- You speak your truth.
- You stand up for yourself.
- You have stronger relationships.
- You laugh more.
- You feel.
- You experience.
- You live the life you've imagined.
- You love yourself.

FREE: OCTOBER 12, 2018

I'm pretty sure that every time I fly I'm going to celebrate the fact that the seatbelt fit and there is even extra strap hanging down. Doing a bit of a happy dance in my head. Woot, woot! I fit in this tiny little seat. Bonus—I can cross my legs!

FAT TO FREE ACTION PLAN

What does success look like for you? Write down at least two sentences to remind yourself how good it will feel to succeed.

This should include tangible items you'll be able to enjoy once you reach your goal. You might say something like "It will feel freeing to be able to shop in all the stores" or "Energy will have me bouncing out of bed in the morning instead of watching life pass by from the couch."

This is a great list to make into a vision board to remind yourself why you are working so hard. It feels good to add check marks or hearts as you accomplish them.

Time to take the great, the good, the bad, the ugly and combine it all into one incredible human being that you genuinely love.

CHAPTER NINETEEN: LOVING YOURSELF

FAT: DECEMBER 7, 2015

I've had great achievements in the last 10 years as a single parent, going back to college and obtaining a wonderful career that keeps me challenged. But even with all of those successes, I don't feel good enough.

The hardest task I had to do to stop my toxic relationship with food was to learn to love myself.

YOU'RE THE KEY

I spent years not feeling good enough for myself or anyone else. I built walls that I thought could never be broken down. Here is what I finally realized: Dwelling on the past or a life challenge is the start of creating excuses. It prevents you from focusing on your priorities. If this journey teaches you anything, I hope you realize it's time to stop hiding behind the lies and excuses that are typically tied to fear.

When I have a task to do, I need to know the reason or the benefit behind it. This chapter includes a surprisingly challenging task—learning to love yourself. I heard it over and over again, but I wasn't sure what it meant or how to get started, so I went looking for information and logic to help me figure it out.

Loving yourself will lead to healthier choices. As you begin to experience success, you'll realize that taking care of yourself is key to continued success. Loving yourself creates this cycle.

Through this process, you'll increase your self-confidence, feel more positive, make choices in line with being healthy, and (one I've enjoyed) worry less about what others think. These may all sound like tall orders, but if you focus on the tools, including learning to love yourself, you'll see that it all happens naturally.

In addition to those benefits, loving yourself is the best, most reliable safety net you have. You always have your own back, your own best interests at heart. As you should! You need to be able to count on yourself when challenges come your way, and the more you face, the stronger you'll be. You're the only one who can make this journey for you.

This topic has been left until the end because I believe it will get the most resistance. At some point, you might have thought, "If I lose the weight, then I will love myself." There are so many attributes we equate with love and value in ourselves. But we've had it backward all this time. Love yourself first and other changes will become easier.

If you loved yourself, do you think you would choose to eat three drive-thru meals while hiding in your car? No! Because people who love and care for themselves make healthy, loving choices for their bodies.

BUILDING SELF-WORTH: LOVING YOUR PAST

How do you define your self-worth? The problem for most of us is that we have been defining it by a number on a scale or the self-declared lack of success in our lives. Success (weight loss) doesn't bring self-love; self-love brings success.

The ultimate self-care step is to embrace and love the person you were when you were overweight. Admittedly, I'm still working on this, but the venture has been one of self-discovery and awareness. I've been extremely hard on myself and the life I lived. I had to accept and embrace that if it weren't for who I was and the choices I made, I wouldn't be where I am today.

Now I love myself and I love my life. I am beyond blessed because of all the challenges I've overcome, and I'm thankful to myself and the life I've lived for getting me here today, sharing with you.

Don't disown who you were—that person got you here. Forgive yourself for any mistakes. You need to love all of you—past, present, and future. It's time to be graceful and accepting of yourself. There's no point in beating yourself up over it. Remember, the real story is how you respond and move forward.

It's also time to trust yourself. Your gut instincts are correct. You know what's best, so stand up for that and protect yourself.

It's sometimes hard to forgive and trust when your past has been filled with years of sadness, loneliness, and anger. But before you fall into guilt and shame, ask yourself this: How is that working for you? Shame, guilt, and disappointment over past choices is only delaying the life you want and have imagined for a long time.

Losing weight comes with many uncomfortable feelings. When you embrace them and push through, it can be unsettling. My life is different than when I started this journey, but I knew it would be. *I wanted it to be.*

No doubt you desire something different as well. For those of us who have tried and failed, there was a missing piece all along. We needed to address our toxic relationship with food. Maybe you didn't know how to stumble and recover. Maybe you're still playing a victim. Maybe it's been all of the above. Now you have the tools. Stop beating yourself up for what you didn't know, and get to work.

You made choices the best way you knew how. Your life led you to right here, and right here is perfect. Your story is powerful and will lead to helping others. Your journey is one you should embrace and respect. Love the person you were, love the person you are now, and love the new person you'll become.

HONEST SELF-REFLECTION: LOVING YOURSELF NOW

Going from fat to free also requires a lot of honest self-reflection. It can be uncomfortable, but it can also be exhilarating. If you haven't said it before, you might be thinking it now: "I don't know who I will be." But since you're already learning how to face fears, figuring out who you are, what you like, and what your priorities are can be some of the most fascinating parts of this process.

I was raised to be a caretaker and a people pleaser. Everyone else's needs were met before mine. It was how I was taught to feel loved. This role played a significant part in my healing. While I was so busy serving others, I had no energy to discover what I enjoyed. I'm learning now. I'm not just talking about whether I like brussels sprouts or hiking (although the answers are no and yes). Today I have values I can confidently, honestly say are all mine—family, honesty, responsibility, commitment, love.

Your acts of self-reflection don't have to be massive; they just have to move you forward. Recently, I tried a hard-boiled egg for the first time. That's right—I'm 50 and never had one before. Hard-boiled eggs are good with hot sauce. I haven't tried deviled eggs yet, but they are on the list.

I find it ridiculous that I had not tried some of these foods before. Now that I'm comfortable being uncomfortable, I try new experiences all the time. I try even when I am scared. Most times, I find it all funny, entertaining, and exciting.

Riding a bike for the first time in so many years was humorous at first because I wobbled so much, but I quickly got the hang of it again and now enjoy riding. Paddleboarding was exciting to the point that I bought my own board and find it a great stress reliever.

Although I am willing to try these new fun activities, I often feel fear when I first try them. I didn't want to fall or jump into the water, because what if I can't get back out? With all of my weight on, I may have been able to physically do it, but I would have been worried that others would laugh at me. It was exciting to jump off my paddleboard and then figure out how to get back on.

I'm no longer just along for the ride. With weight loss came confidence. And now that I have more confidence, I've realized that I don't want to follow along and live my life based on what everyone else chooses.

One of my favorite parts of this journey was letting go of what other people think of me. I strongly suggest you do the same. What others think is their opinion and that's all. People judge. People have opinions. But if you're wasting your time concerned with what other people think of you, your mind is going into a negative space and wasting your time and energy, which could be better spent advancing your own healing.

Trust me, this is coming from a woman who lived 30+ years of her life worrying about what others thought. Most of my worrying about others' opinions was centered around me being overweight. Like what if my fat hung over the table in a booth? What if I couldn't keep up with my walking partner?

There is no benefit to worrying about what others think. Why spend energy on what you cannot control? Detach from what others think of you. The reality is that not everyone is going to like you no matter what you do, and those thoughts they have about you are more about them anyway.

It is hard to let go, but stop pursuing the belief that if you get things right, you will be loved and admired. Practice feeling good and confident about yourself. You have strength—use it to focus on loving yourself and your journey. Find your tribe of people who love you for who you are and keep them close.

LIGHT YOUR FIRE: LOVE YOUR POSSIBILITY

It's time to take your flicker of hope and desire and light it on fire, turn it on bright. It's your turn to shine.

You have a fire within you. It may be a small spark, but it's there, and it's time to make it into a roaring fire. It can start with any small thought going through your head. You've got to catch it and build on it.

Maybe you're driving, hear a good song, and think, *I wish I could play that on the piano.*

Or you're dropping your kids off at school and think, *I wish I had the nerve to volunteer in my kid's class.*

Maybe you're sitting on the couch while everyone else is out riding bikes or playing in the snow and you think, *I wish I had the energy to join in.*

Or you're at work, hear about a promotion, and think, *I wish I were good enough to go for it.*

To identify your fire, you just have to start paying attention. What happens each day that has you sitting back and daydreaming of possibilities? If you desire something different than what you're doing right now, that's it. We all have one.

You survived. You're here. You're unique. You're worthy. You're loveable.

By loving yourself unconditionally, you'll find the courage and strength to discover your light, build your fire, and live free.

BREAKING UP WITH YOURSELF

When I had reached my goal weight, I was talking with a friend about our recent breakups. She shared an exercise she had done to move on from her romantic relationship, and we realized it would also be helpful for ending a toxic relationship with food.

In a sense, you "break up" with yourself, noting all the qualities you didn't like from your former life, then detailing how you wish to be going forward.

Here are some examples of what you might say.

I didn't like...

>...how my body felt after eating an enormous amount of food.
>
>...how I couldn't wear cute clothes or shoes.
>
>...how round my face was.
>
>...sweating profusely when I hardly moved.
>
>...taking six medications.
>
>...always feeling exhausted.
>
>...feeling like a failure.

What I do like is...

>...choosing to fuel my body properly
>
>...going shopping and fitting in clothes that are smaller sizes.
>
>...how slim my face looks now (with only one chin!).
>
>...being comfortable at all different temperatures.

...saving money on medications and doctor appointments.

...having energy for the entire day.

...feeling confident.

FREE: JUNE 7, 2020

Feeling my emotions is still unfamiliar at times, but I continue to embrace it more each day.

I stumbled today. I struggled today. I didn't eat those feelings, but I felt them. I cried. I let go.

Life is hard, but I'm okay. I am Elizabeth and I love myself.

YOUR LESSON:
Learn to love yourself.

FAT TO FREE ACTION PLAN

1. Write a list of reasons you want to break up with your old self. List the old habits, feelings, and negative aspects that you're happy to leave in the past. Write down anything that reminds

you of where you have been and where you don't want to go again.

2. Then write out a positive description of where you want to be.

Remember that breaking up with your old self doesn't negate the love. Break up, forgive, and move on. Moving on can get stalled by all the what-if scenarios we come up with. But remember, they are fear based.

Are you still on the fence about making changes? Here comes a little more incentive.

CHAPTER TWENTY: JUMPING IN

FAT: JUNE 23, 2007

Sitting at the pool. Feeling gross and uncomfortable in my bathing suit. Trying not to care about my body and how fat I feel. Was doing okay until Sophie's friend showed up with her dad. I have always liked him from far away but have never said anything. I'm burning up and just want to get in the pool, but there's no way I'm going to walk in front of him!

SITTING ON THE SIDELINES

How is it possible I ever looked in a mirror or saw pictures of my fat self and could still convince myself that nobody noticed my size? I spent years avoiding mirrors, cameras, my reflection, and even my shadow. If I didn't see myself, they couldn't either, right? I felt shame and sadness, but somehow I'd spend each day believing that if I wore big clothes, stayed out of photos, and blocked out my reality, no one would notice me. I didn't really want to notice myself either.

My denial reached a new peak one day at the neighborhood pool when I tried to plot how I could get from my lounge chair into the water without drawing any attention. I remember thinking that if I could just get in the water, I'd be totally hidden. Now I consider myself a smart woman, but lady—water is clear!

You may think you're hiding, but everyone can see you.

Approximately 15 years ago, I was a single mom, going to school and working full time. I was the fattest I had ever been. I don't know how big, because I didn't step on a scale unless I was at the doctor's office. And even then, I'd just look away.

Sophie and I lived in nice little home in a great neighborhood with a pool. I enjoyed taking her swimming. It provided an opportunity for her to have fun with her friends and I could sit close by. Simply by sitting there, being out in the sun and spending time with my daughter, I felt less guilty than if I had been at home on the couch.

During our walk to the pool one day, Sophie asked, "Mom, are you getting in today?"

I replied, "I'm not sure yet."

The truth was that I needed to scope out who was there before deciding whether I'd remove my cover-up and expose my fat body.

Sitting on the side of the pool is like sitting on the sidelines of life. I chose sidelines over and over, but I really wanted to swim with my daughter. It's why I wrapped my body in a big, black bathing suit. But the suit never hid the fat the way I wished it would.

On this particular day, Sophie was in the pool and I was on a chair staring down at my phone and avoiding any potential eye contact.

Sophie called out, "Hey, Mom—are you going to get in the pool and play with me?"

My reply was almost always the same. "I can't right now, sweetie. I have to finish these messages." I had endless ways to say no.

Sophie would look at me, disappointed and sad. Eventually she stopped asking.

On the day I described in my journal entry above, the guy was the cute dad of Sophie's friend who lived down the street. There was no way I was going to let him see me in my bathing suit. That day was miserably hot. I was sweating and uncomfortable. The plastic-strap lounge chair was sticking to my legs. The sound it made when I moved was awful. I wondered how far the straps had stretched under my large body.

That day, I wrote in my journal how desperately I wanted to find the strength to get out of the chair. "Why am I such a chickenshit that I can't get up off this chair and into the pool? I'm missing out!"

My promise to consider getting in the pool with Sophie quickly became no option at all when her friend's dad arrived. I had been crushing on him since we met, and I saw him often because our girls were friends. It was never more than casual greetings, then daydreams about what it would be like for him to ask me out.

What if he notices I'm fat?

What if he hears the noise my legs make peeling off the chair?

What if he sees sweat dripping down my back?

What if he talks to me?

What if he laughs at me?

Sophie splashed in the pool with her friend. I made an excuse and stayed on the sidelines. I stayed in the chair and hid. My daughter swam alone. This man was always kind and would say hello. I threw a towel over me while we chatted. We would make plans for the next time our girls would get together, and then he would get in the pool and have fun with them.

GET IN THE GAME

Life now is very different. But here I am at the end of my forties and single again. The dating world is far different than it was 10 years ago. Everybody's jumping online and downloading apps to meet new people. You have to decide whether you'll swipe right or swipe left. Who do you wink at? When do you boost your like? When you match, do you message first? The options are seemingly endless—in terms of both communication styles and men.

My friends felt that I needed a nudge to get back out there and start letting go of the past. They helped me create a profile on a few different sites. We uploaded pictures and added descriptions and, before I knew it, I was starting to swipe. I wasn't prepared for the amount of time online dating takes.

One day, I was checking my notifications when up popped his picture. That's right: the pool dad. He was single and looking. I romanticized what an incredible story this would be. But in that same moment, I started to what-if the situation.

What if he doesn't remember me?

What if he doesn't respond?

What if he does?

What if we go out and I make a fool of myself on the date?

What if he always liked me too?

I started sharing the story with others, and my friends encouraged me to do what I had planned to do already.

I swiped right. And we matched! I sent a message and even took it one step further by asking him out. When I go bold, I don't hold back. After all, this was going to be my fairy-tale ending. I was excited and curious. I wondered how long it would take him to respond. What would he say?

I'd check every so often to see if he had read the message. The day passed and my excitement started to wear off. Later that night, I checked again. He had read my message...several hours ago. He never did respond.

Sometimes you win, sometimes you lose. Sometimes things just aren't meant to be. Sure it's fun to daydream from time to time, but what matters is that you don't let life pass you by while you're living in fear of the what-ifs. Better to just jump in and see.

I jumped in, and I survived. I had my tools handy. I didn't need anyone else's validation. I put myself out there, and I was proud of that. I have continued to swipe right, like, and chat with others. Though my heart has not yet found a new connection, I am having fun dating. No regrets.

I'm not sure whether it was because of my weight loss or the fact that I'm in my late forties (most likely a combination of both), but I finally got myself up off the sidelines. I jumped in the pool. I'm playing the game. I don't care what others think. I no longer dodge photos, mirrors, or my shadow. It didn't happen overnight.

I trained myself to see the real me. I worked at it. And it changed my life.

Are you a what-if-er? Before you take any action, you analyze the decision into the ground. You look at every possible angle of how it may turn out.

What if I say the wrong thing?

What if I don't get the job?

What if it doesn't work this time?

What if I fail?

What if nobody reads my book?

That's right, I know all of them from experience.

Now here we are. You have all the tools to be successful on your journey, but you might still be what-if-ing your choice to go from fat to free.

Look in the mirror and start to accept yourself, no matter your size. Anyone worthy of being in your life doesn't care about your size, especially your family, close friends, and loved ones. They care about you, your time, and your love. Share those things with them.

I imagine that through many of the chapters you read in this book, especially the last one, your negative voice was trying to be loud. Your brain thought of excuses as you read my ideas. You might still feel that I don't understand your struggles. That I just got lucky.

It doesn't matter what those voices try to tell you; what matters is that you love yourself enough to push past that negativity and start making positive choices.

It's time to act. Reading this book is only the beginning. Writing in your journal is just a first step. Make the decision to change your life and take action now. Yes, it will be hard, but I promise you it will be worth it. The journey is beautiful. It will include so much more than a number on the scale.

So stop asking questions and coming up with excuses. This is your time.

You're worthy.

I believe in you.

I love you.

Choose you!

FREE: OCTOBER 19, 2019

Oh my goodness. Did I just do that? Yep, I did. The fear was present. The fear was pushed aside. I took a leap of faith. This girl is going after what she wants.

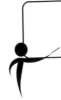

> **YOUR LESSON:**
> *Choose you.*

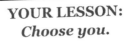

FAT TO FREE ACTION PLAN

Throughout this book, you've created many tools and lists. As a review, I want you to revisit four of them that you'll use every day. Write out each of the four items below again in your journal. Update them if necessary.

1. Chapter Two > Your Why

2. Chapter Four > Your Goal

3. Chapter Sixteen > Your Affirmations

4. Chapter Eighteen > Your Vision

Make copies and put them on the fridge, on the mirror in the bathroom, by the bed, in the living room, in your car, in your purse, and in your office. Add pictures or quotes of items that remind you about your why. Make it fun and colorful so it catches your eye. When you feel the desire to reach for food rather than take care of yourself, this will be a powerful visual reminder.

CHAPTER TWENTY-ONE: THEN WHAT?

FAT: JUNE 14, 2007

I cried. I let myself feel the pain, and I'm going to continue to let myself feel it.

ENDLESS OPPORTUNITIES

I knew I needed to feel my pain, but I rarely documented it in my journal. I cried often. I wept out of anger, frustration, and embarrassment, usually because I was afraid. Fear was front and center. For a long time, it stopped me from trying new things and taking steps to better my life. Friends would see my fear, call it out, and try to open my eyes to the fact that most times I had built it up into something larger than it needed to be.

In the last chapter, you learned about what-ifs. Have you ever played the game "Then what?" Whenever my friend and I are uncertain about something, we play it. It works for simple decisions or more difficult emotionally charged ones.

It's pretty simple. You state what you're considering and the other person asks, "Then what?"

You do this to expose all the possible outcomes—good or bad—that could happen. This exercise helps you understand whenever your hesitation, which is most likely out of fear, is unwarranted. List them all, even the highly unlikely. Find the opportunity. Realize that each answer to "Then what?" is just the beginning of another question. Asking that keeps you moving forward, even over hypothetical stumbles.

For example, if you said, "I am thinking about quitting my job," your partner would ask, "Then what?" You then list all the possible awful or wonderful things that could happen. As you do this, two things happen. The first is that you realize there aren't really that many and that some of them are just ridiculous. The second is that you generally get through to the good stuff pretty quickly, likely even with some laughter. Have fun with it too, because as you have read, humor is always helpful.

Some possible scenarios could be...

"My colleagues will never talk to me again."

"Then what?"

"I'll have more energy and focus to give to my real support network."

"No one will want to hire me."

"Then what?"

~~~

"I'll work on my hobbies or personal projects I've been putting off. I'll take classes to become more marketable and spend my energy networking."

"I'll find a better job that makes me feel more fulfilled and even pays more."

"Then what?"

"I'll feel challenged, respected, and accomplished."

Do you see how that goes? What-ifs are a dead end; "Then what?" creates endless opportunities.

So you're coming to the end of the book. You have the tools and the knowledge. It's time to take action. Scared? Let's play "Then what?"

> You say, "I'm going to start taking steps to end my toxic relationship with food."
>
> And I ask, "Then what?"
>
> "I will feel uncomfortable."
>
> "Then what?"
>
> "I will learn skills that help me navigate life challenges even when I am uncomfortable."
>
> "Then what?"
>
> "It will be hard."
>
> "Then what?"
>
> "I will still be successful because I have survived other difficult situations in my life."
>
> "Then what?"

"I might fail."

"Then what?"

"I might far exceed my own expectations."

"Then what?"

"I'll keep going."

"Then what?"

"I'll reach my goal!"

You could do this all day and it will always have the same ending. But you're strong and have already done so much hard work. You've been down this path so many times before. And now you have the tools and solutions to end your toxic relationship with food.

FINDING LIGHTNESS

Reminisce about when you were a kid. You would play with your friends all day and the only thing you had to worry about was being home on time. Or how about riding a bike? Or riding in a car with the windows rolled down? Do you remember the wind blowing your hair? Hanging your hand out and letting the wind push it up and down? Your hair in your face, the music pumping, you are singing and feeling at peace, full of energy and ready to tackle the world.

Being free of my fat is like that feeling multiplied by 100. I am lighter than I've ever been before, feel like I can tackle anything. My fear and anxiety have lessened. I no longer watch others doing all the things I want to do; I'm doing them. I no longer drag myself out of bed but rather jump up, ready to take on the world.

Being free of the physical weight and mentally free of worry and anxiety is a blessing. Being in control of how to fuel my body properly is beautiful. After two years, I'm still shocked at the amount of free time I have because I'm no longer obsessing over what I look like. I no longer care what others think about me. The weight is off my body and off my mind, and I feel new, blessed, joyful, peaceful, and free!

Cherish your memories of the past, but put your energy into what is to come and not on what is lost. All the pain, challenges, and sadness have a purpose you probably can't see yet. You've been through difficult times.

You deserve this. You're worthy! You can have all the experiences that you desire.

Choose to go from fat to free.

FREE: MARCH 1, 2020

My life was full of beauty, but it is even more beautiful now. Finishing this book is one of the freest moments I've ever had. As I sit here with a completed manuscript, I find it hard to express what I'm feeling. Confident. Excited. Blessed. Happy. Ready. The world in all of its obstacles, sadness, and hardships is beautiful, and I believe I have so much more to do.

FAT TO FREE ACTION PLAN

Here is a summary of the lists you made that will support you on your journey, in priority order.

- ◊ The Big Four: your why, your goal, your affirmations, your vision for success (Chapter Twenty)
- ◊ Your priorities and values (Chapter Eight)
- ◊ Your break-up list (Chapter Nineteen)
- ◊ Strategies to protect yourself (Chapter Eleven)
- ◊ Your emergency and travel plan (Chapter Five)
- ◊ Responses to stumbles (Chapter Fifteen)
- ◊ Experiences and rewards instead of food (Chapter Thirteen)

So the only thing left you for you to do is answer this question: Then what?

Take some time to reflect on what comes next for you in your journal.

LESSONS LEARNED

◊ Always come back to your why. (Chapter One)

◊ Identify your emotional eating as it's happening. Call it what it is. (Chapter Two)

◊ Own your choices. (Chapter Three)

◊ Have realistic expectations. (Chapter Four)

◊ Stop being a victim. (Chapter Five)

◊ Set goals and objectives. Find appropriate rewards. (Chapter Six)

◊ Recognize when you're hungry. Recognize when you're full. (Chapter Seven)

◊ Stop making excuses and sabotaging your own life. (Chapter Eight)

◊ Be vulnerable, present your true self, and build your support system. (Chapter Nine)

◊ Stop lying to yourself. (Chapter Ten)

◊ Break your bad habits. Build new ones. Actively protect yourself, your goals, and your health. (Chapter Eleven)

◊ Face your fears. (Chapter Twelve)

◊ Be comfortable being uncomfortable. (Chapter Thirteen)

- ◊ Use a scale to listen to your body. (Chapter Fourteen)

- ◊ Learn from your stumbles. (Chapter Fifteen)

- ◊ Learn to use affirmations. (Chapter Sixteen)

- ◊ Practice all six areas of self-care. (Chapter Seventeen)

- ◊ Know that your journey doesn't end when you reach your goal weight. Face your fears and celebrate your blessings. (Chapter Eighteen)

- ◊ Learn to love yourself. (Chapter Nineteen)

- ◊ Choose you. (Chapter Twenty)

REFERENCES

"Are You a Food Addict?" Quiz. FoodAddicts.org. https://www.foodaddicts.org/am-i-a-food-addict.

Carlson, Richard. *Don't Sweat the Small Stuff*. Hachette Books, 1997.

Clear, James. *Atomic Habits*. Avery, 2018.

Clough, Joseph. "Hypnosis With Joseph Clough." App. https://www.josephclough.com/apps/ios, https://www.josephclough.com/android-free-hypnosis-app.

Dominee. "Types of Self-Care You Need to Know." BlessingManifesting.com. https://www.blessingmanifesting.com/2017/07/what-is-self-care.html.

Haden, Jeff. "Change Any Habit Painlessly: 6 Tips." Inc.com. https://www.inc.com/jeff-haden/change-any-habit-painlessly-6-tips.html.

Hernandez, Wendy. "12 Reasons You Should Never Regret Any Decision You Ever Make." Lifehack.org. https://www.lifehack.org/articles/communication/12-reasons-you-should-never-regret-any-decision-you-ever-make.html.

Hyman, Mark. Twitter Post. July 13, 2020, 3:00 p.m. https://twitter.com/drmarkhyman/status/1282751789922648065.

Stöppler, Melissa Conrad. "Medical Definition of Emotional eating." MedicineNet.com. https://www.medicinenet.com/script/main/art.asp?articlekey=46450.

RECOMMENDED
RESOURCES

Atomic Habits. An Easy & Proven Way to Build Good Habits & Break Bad Ones by James Clear

Better Human: It's a Full-Time Job by Ronda Conger

The Code Red Revolution by Cristy "Code Red" Nickel

Don't Sweat the Small Stuff...and It's All Small Stuff by Richard Carlson

Extreme Ownership: How U.S. Navy SEALs Lead and Win by Jocko Willink and Leif Babin

Relationship Development, Stacey & Paul Martino, relationshipdevelopment.org

*Unfu*k Yourself: Get Out of Your Head and Into Your Life* by Gary John Bishop

Unstoppable Influence by Natasha Hazlett

ACKNOWLEDGMENTS

For anyone who is reading this and has been a part of my story, I love you more than myself. I have great memories. I have amazing stories. There was laughter. There was goodness. You were blessings in my life. Those of you who are still in my life will forever be held in my heart as people who loved me no matter what. Thank you!

Jamie, you always ask, and I have been able to count on that for more than 30 years. You lifted me up at a time that most would have backed off due to their own pain. You didn't. Thank you!

KC, thank you for supporting me and, most importantly, understanding what I'm saying when half the time I'm not even sure. You take my random thoughts, ideas, and requests and turn them into workable and professional content that keeps this project moving forward. I can't wait to see where we are in the next year.

My Camp Rainbow Gold family, you have inspired and held me up on some of the most difficult days of my life. Together we have experienced sadness but also a great deal of joy, laughter, and love. Being a part of a group that truly leads through life with kindness and compassion has helped me stay focused and determined to keep leveling up what I bring each day. Thank you to each of you for being such a blessing in my life.

Cristy "Code Red," Cari Thompson, and all of the Code Red staff, leaders, and coaches—thank you for introducing me to a new lifestyle and not just another diet. Learning how to properly fuel my body with real foods was the first step for me to finally lose weight. I couldn't have done it without the program Cristy developed, or without the unprecedented support that came with it. Not only did you teach me how to live the lifestyle, you have also entrusted me to teach others and be a force to change lives to help get our world healthy.

Natasha and Rich Hazlett, your teaching led me to the missing link I had been searching for. Thank you for showing me how to embrace being perfectly imperfect, which helped me discover how to stop emotional eating. I'll never forget sitting in your summit when I was still in the early stages of this process and writing the words "I will write a book." Who knew you would be publishing it!

ABOUT THE AUTHOR

Elizabeth has survived a 35-year battle with health, weight loss, and a toxic relationship with food. Now she is sharing her journey to life 100 pounds lighter in the hope that even just one person with weight to lose will know they are not alone.

Elizabeth applies her natural inclination to help others and her acute business acumen in many aspects of her life. She is the CEO of Camp Rainbow Gold, a nonprofit serving children who have been diagnosed with cancer. She was an *Idaho Business Review* Women of the Year nominee in 2014 and was recognized as a CEO of Influence in 2017. Though the recognition is appreciated, her greatest joy is seeing the impact her work has on the lives of others.

Elizabeth lives in Boise, Idaho, and is a mother to Sophie and her bonus kids, Kenny and Katie. She enjoys getting outdoors to ride her bike, hike, and go paddleboarding. You can continue to follow Elizabeth's journey and join the conversation at www.FromFatToFree.com.

Email: elizabeth@FromFattoFree.com

Facebook: @fromfat2free

Instagram: @fromfat_tofree

LinkedIn: From Fat to Free, Elizabeth Lizberg

YouTube: From Fat to Free

Made in the USA
Monee, IL
27 July 2021

74353947R10134